Beyond Antibiotics: Exploring Host-Directed Therapy for TB

Jessy

Table of Contents

Chapter 1: Introduction and Literature review 2

1.1 Introduction 2

1.2 Background 2

1.3 Long non-coding RNAs 4

1.4 lncRNA classification and characteristic features 6

1.5 Mechanism of action of lncRNAs 7

1.6 LncRNAs in host–pathogen interactions 8

1.7 ncRNAs regulate the innate immune system 9

1.7.1 *LincRNA-Cox2* facilitates the induction and repression of gene expression in mouse macrophages 9

1.7.2 *THRIL* regulates TNF-α release and global gene expression in human monocytic THP-1 cells 10

1.7.3 lincRNA-EPS regulates the expression of immune response genes in macrophages. 10

1.7.4 lncRNA Mirt2 is a negative regulator of inflammation 11

1.8 Functionally validated lncRNAs during Mtb infection 11

1.8.1 lncRNA-CD244 epigenetically controls CD8+ T-cell immune responses in tuberculosis infection. 11

1.8.2 The antituberculosis effect of lncRNA NEAT1 12

1.8.3 The role of lncRNA PCED1B-AS1 12

1.9 Functionally validated lncRNAs in *Mycobacterium bovis* BCG 12

1.9.1 LncRNA MEG3 eradicates mycobacteria in macrophages via autophagy 12

1.9.2 lincRNA-Cox2 induces intracellular mycobacterium killing in macrophages 12

1.10 Expression profiles of lncRNAs in immune cells infected with Mtb 13

1.11 Differential expression of lncRNAs in serum, active TB vs healthy or latent individuals 13

1.12 LncRNA interaction 13

1.12.1 LncRNAs and gene interaction 13

1.12.2 lncRNAs and protein interaction 14

1.12.3 lncRNAs and disease association 14

1.13 lncRNA bioinformatics 15

1.13.1 LncRNAs secondary and tertiary structures 15

1.13.2 Computational prediction of ncRNA secondary structure... 15

1.13.3 Computational prediction of ncRNA tertiary structure 15

1.14 The role of lincRNA-MIR99AHG in cancer 16

1.14.1 MIR99AHG and MIR100HG act as oncogenes in acute megakaryoblastic leukemia (AMKL) 16

1.15 Possible proximal genes adjacent to MIR99AHG gene 16

1.15.1 Cxadr 16

1.15.2 Usp25 17

1.15.3 Bach1 17

1.15.4 Btg3 17

1.16 Host-directed therapy as adjunct therapy 18

1.17 Antisense oligonucleotide delivery 19

1.18 FDA approved ASOs and ASOs in clinical trials 20

1.19 Research problem and focus... 20

1.20 Aim... 21

1. 20.1 The objectives of the study: 21

1.21 Hypothesis 21

Chapter 2: Materials and Methods... 21

2.1 Materials.. 21

2.2 Methods... 21

2.2.1 Ethics Statement 21

2.2.2 Generation of Bone Marrow-Derived Macrophages (BMDMs) 22

2.2.3 Generation of peripheral blood mononuclear cells (PBMCs) and monocyte-derived macrophages (MDMs).. 22

2.2.4 Culture of RAW264.7 murine macrophage cell line... 23

2.2.5 Transfection of BMDMs and MDMs 23

2.2.6 Stimulation and *Mycobacterium tuberculosis* infection of BMDMs and MDMs 23

2.2.7 RNA Extraction 23

2.2.8 cDNA Synthesis and RT-qPCR... 24

2.2.9 Bacterial Burden Determination.. 24

2.2.10 Cytokine Production... 24

2.2.11 Griess reagent assay.. 24

2.2.12 Arginase assay 24

2.2.13 RNA pull-down assay 25

2.2.14 RNA Immunoprecipitation (RIP)... 25

2.2.15 Western blot..25

2.2.16 RNA sequencing and data analysis 25

2.2.17 *In vivo* GapmeR challenge..26

2.2.18 Histology...26

2.2.19 Flow cytometry..26

2.2.20 Mtb infection and determination of burdens in mice 26

2.2.21 Cell viability and apoptosis 26

2.2.22 Statistical analysis 27

Chapter 3: Mtb targets lincRNA-MIR99AHG for evasion in macrophages.........................28

3.1 Introduction...28

3.2 Results 30

3.2.1 MIR99AHG is induced by IL-4/IL-13 and repressed by Mtb HN878 infection 30

3.2.2 Knockdown of MIR99AHG reduces intracellular Mtb growth and inflammatory cytokines
....32

3.2.3 *Cis*-acting MIR99AHG regulates the expression of nearby gene, Cxadr...........................35

3.2.4 *In vivo* treatment with LNA GapmeRs for MIR99AHG reduced mycobacterial burden in
mice..38

3.2.5 MIR99AHG leads to TB disease progression by inducing pro-inflammatory responses in
the lung macrophages...41

3.2.6 MIR99AHG is repressed in macrophages exposed to TLR ligands and its expression is
dependent on IL-4Rα signalling 43

3.2.7 MIR99AHG is translocated from the cytoplasm to the nucleus following IL-4/IL-13
stimulation in macrophages and functions by interacting with hnRNPA2/B1 45

3.2.8 Suppression of MIR99AHG in Mtb-infected human macrophages and active TB patients
....47

3.3 Discussion 49

3.4 Conclusion 53

3.5 Supplementary figures 54

Chapter 4: IL7-AS promotes Mtb intracellular growth through regulation of inflammatory genes .59

4.1 Introduction...59

4.2 Results 60

4.2.1 IL7-AS is induced following Mtb infection...60

4.2.2 Knockdown of IL7-AS reduces intracellular Mtb growth through apoptosis and
regulation of the transcription of inflammatory genes 61

4.2.3 IL7-AS functions independently of IL-7...63

4.2.4 IL7-AS is induced in Mtb infected mice 67

4.2.5 IL7-AS is induced in BMDMs exposed to TLR ligands and dependent on the Myd88
signalling pathway..67

4.2.6 IL7-AS is induced in Mtb-infected human macrophages and active TB patients 70

4.3 Discussion 72

Chapter 5: General discussion and conclusions 76

5.1 Aim for chapter 3 76

5.2 Summary of results from Chapter 3 76

5.3 Studies contributing to generation of the hypothesis in Chapter 3 77

5.4 Conclusions to Chapter 3 77

5.5 Aim for chapter 4 78

5.6 Summary of results from chapter 4 78

5.7 Studies contributing to generation of the hypothesis in Chapter 4 78

5.8 Conclusion to Chapter 4 79

5.9 Relevance of studies and future work 79

References 80

Chapter 1: Introduction and Literature review
1.1 Introduction
Tuberculosis (TB), caused by *Mycobacterium tuberculosis* (Mtb), is one of the leading infectious diseases in the world [1]. Globally, 1.7 billion people are infected with Mtb and are at risk of developing active tuberculosis [1] It is estimated that TB causes more than 1.5 million deaths per year with Africa experiencing the second highest burden (24%) [1]. The eight countries which contributed the most to the global disease burden included South Africa [1]. There is an urgent need to develop new treatment approaches due to the rise of multi-drug resistant strains of TB, the amount of time required to complete treatment and some factors that cause patients not to complete treatment. South Africa has one of the highest burdens of TB cases which may lead to a multi-drug epidemic [2]. Novel anti-TB therapies need to be developed as more research identifies important crucial factors that play a role in the pathogenesis of TB. There is growing awareness towards host factors and one of the recent approaches is to develop host-directed therapy (HDT) [3]. Host directed therapeutics targets host responses that Mtb may hijack to induce persistence within the host rather than targeting the pathogen directly by conventional antibiotics. Targeting HDT results in a reduction in pathology, mycobacterial burden and possible latency that could be achieved by targeting and using the same host factors Mtb uses [3]. For countries such as South Africa which face an epidemic of multi-drug resistant TB, targeting host factors as therapy is less likely to cause multi-drug resistance compared to the FDA-approved drugs. For host-directed targets to be effective they must be able to induce a variety of host-pathogen protective mechanisms such as the innate signalling pathway, phagosomal maturation, bactericidal mechanisms, autophagy, prevent Mtb binding and uptake, phagosomal escape and/or detoxification [4]. However, Mtb has evolved mechanisms in which it is able to prevent inhibition of phagosomal acidification by inhibition of proton ATPase [5], preventing calcium signalling [6] and hindering the fusion machinery of vesicular transport [7].

1.2 Background
Mtb is predominantly transmitted by the respiratory route, and while it is able to cause disease in most organs in the body, the most reported and occurring is pulmonary tuberculosis [8]. The host immune response against Mtb infection is complex and multifaceted. The GENCODE project, with the aim to show all functional importance in human DNA, estimates that 2% of the mammalian genome comprises of protein-coding genes while

98% is transcribed as non-coding RNAs [9]. Non-coding RNAs (ncRNA) are mainly categorized as either short ncRNA (<200 nucleotides) or long ncRNA (>200 nucleotides) [10]. Very little is known about long noncoding RNAs (lncRNAs) and their functions. Recent published research now shows that lncRNAs play a significant role in many physiological and pathological processes [11]. The function of lncRNAs in immune cells is recently emerging [12]. A few studies have been conducted to demonstrate lncRNA function in immune cells. For example, *lincRNA-EPS* is an inhibitor of immune response gene (IRG) expression, acting as a regulatory checkpoint that is downregulated prior to inducible expression of IRGs [13]. Many other lncRNAs including *lincRNA-Cox2* [14], *THRIL* [15], *Mirt2* [16], and *lnc13* [17] also regulate inflammatory genes in myeloid cells.

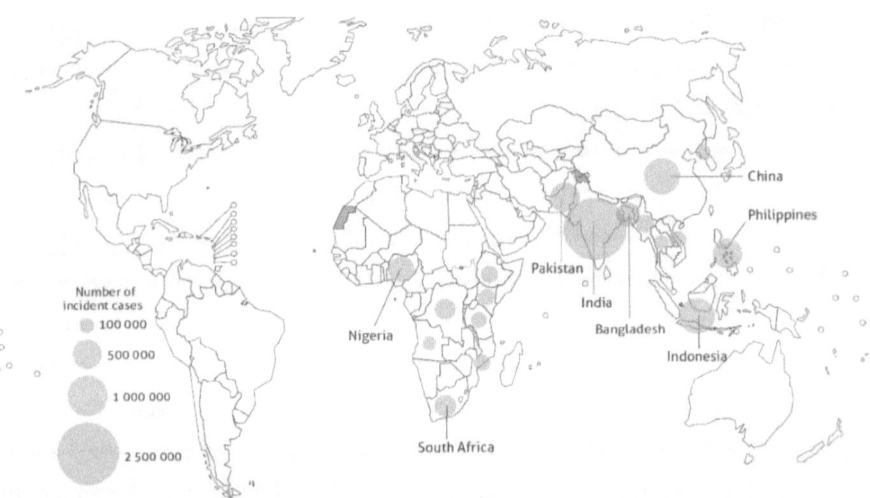

Figure 1.1 Estimated countries with highest TB incidence. Image sourced form WHO [1].

There is very limited work on functionally validated lncRNAs in response to Mtb infection and no scientific research/publication of functionally validated lncRNAs in polarised M1 (IFNγ) or M2 (IL-4/IL-13) and/or Mtb infected macrophages. Due to the lack of limited research on the role of lncRNAs during Mtb infection we sought to identify the functional role of lincRNA-

MIR99AHG in polarised Mtb-infected macrophages and its prophylactic effect on Mtb-infected mice.

1.3 Long non-coding RNAs

The activation of the innate and adaptive immune cells cannot be induced without a coordinated set of transcriptional and post transcriptional events [18]. During these events many protein-coding genes are activated and repressed [18]. A potential host-derived drug target which has recently gained awareness is long non-coding RNAs (lncRNA). Both DNA strands are generally transcribed, which then gives rise to many various classes of non-coding RNAs (ncRNAs) [19]. Approximately 167 150 and 130 558 lncRNA transcripts have been identified in humans and mice, respectively [20]. There are many different expression patterns of lncRNAs in various cell types, tissues, developmental stages, and context-specific manners [21]. This abundant mixture of long and short non-coding RNAs was misunderstood in past years as transcriptional noise or junk [22].

Very little is known about lncRNAs although, in comparison with miRNAs, these are generally shorter in length, contain fewer albeit longer exons, and are expressed at lower levels [22-24]. lncRNAs are poorly conserved, with an estimation of only 15% of mouse protein coding genes reported to have human homologues, leading to assumption that the many lncRNAs are not functional [24-27]. Currently, lncRNAs are arranged according to their position relative to protein-coding genes [10]. These include the long intergenic ncRNA (lincRNAs) located between protein coding genes, intronic lncRNAs which are transcribed from intronic regions in either sense or antisense orientation, antisense lncRNAs which are transcribed across the exons of protein coding genes, transcribed pseudogene lncRNAs, bidirectional lncRNAs which are located on the opposite strand from a protein coding gene and enhancer RNA (eRNAs), which are less than 2 kb in length, these are bidirectionally transcribed from enhancer regions [10]. There is increasing research on the function and mechanism of lncRNAs, this includes chromatin modification, transcriptional regulation, post transcriptional regulation and gene regulation [10]. LncRNAs have been reported to be important regulators of physiological and pathological responses [11, 28]. However, their importance in the innate immune response is only now becoming prominent. A few studies have been conducted on the functional role of lncRNAs in the immune system. This literature review will investigate functions of how lncRNAs regulate the innate immune system specifically during bacterial infection, host-pathogen interaction, their mechanism of action and how we identified lincRNA-MIR99AHG.

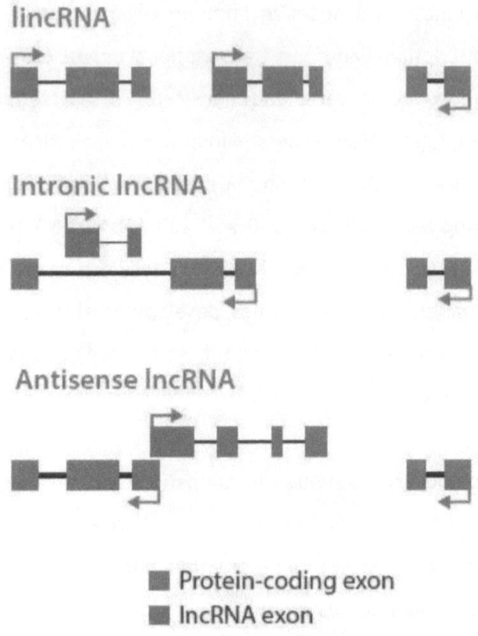

Figure 1.2 Classification of lncRNAs based on their genomic location with respect to nearby protein-coding genes. Image sourced from Atianand *et al*. [12].

FANTOM (Functional Annotation Of the Mammalian genome) is an international research consortium developed by RIKEN mainly centred on functional annotation of mammalian genomes and characterization of transcriptional regulatory networks. The FANTOM5 consortium, with over 500 international members from 20 countries, has generated maps of human regulatory elements and transcriptional regulatory network models. To attain this goal, they used CAGE (Cap Analysis of Gene Expression) sequencing on RNA samples from every major human organs, various primary cell types, over 200 cancer cell lines, 30 time courses of cellular differentiation, and mouse developmental time courses.

Using the CAGE approach, 64 lncRNA transcripts that were differentially expressed upon cytokine stimulation and/or Mtb infection on BMDMs were identified. The selected lncRNAs were either induced upon M1 (IFN-γ), M2 (IL-4, IL-13) or Mtb stimulation. Subsequent RT-qPCR validation yielded a shortlist of 9 lncRNAs on M1 and M2 polarised macrophages which we intend on functionally validating. Five lncRNAs encoded by the same phylogenetically well conserved gene, the MIR99AHG gene, were highly induced by IL-4/IL-13. The analysis of the MIR99AHG gene locus showed enrichment and overlapping of H3K4m1, H3K4me3 and H3K27ac marks; CTCF and POLII binding on the first exon of those lncRNAs, indicative of an active transcription and a potential enhancer-like function. There has been one study conducted on MIR99AHG wherein MIR99AHG and MIR100HG have been shown to act as ancogenes in acute megakaryoblastic leukaemia [29]. We also chose to functionally validate IL7-AS which was highly upregulated upon Mtb infection. There is increasing literature describing the functional role of IL7-AS in biological processes [30, 31] but limited research on its role during Mtb infection. Due to limited research on the effect of lncRNA regulation in polarized macrophages and during Mtb infection, we sought to establish the functional role of MIR99AHG and IL7-AS in polarized macrophages and during Mtb infection.

1.4 lncRNA classification and characteristic features

Approximately 2% of the human genome is transcribed into protein-coding RNAs, the remaining 98% is transcribed into non protein-coding RNAs referred to as non-coding RNAs (ncRNAs) [32]. These ncRNAs include many types of RNA. Examples include transfer RNAs (tRNAs), ribosomal RNAs (rRNAs) and small nuclear RNAs (snRNAs), with well-defined functions in various cellular processes [33-36]. There are other various ncRNAs with unknown functions and limited information, many of which are considered as lncRNAs [33, 37]. These lncRNAs are poorly conserved and are distinguished by their positions respective to the protein-coding genes [10, 37, 38]. They have some similarities with protein-coding transcripts; in general these lncRNAs are transcribed by the RNA polymerase II and can be capped, polyadenylated and spliced [32]. The lncRNAs are either localized in the nucleus or the cytoplasm [34].

Currently lncRNAs are classified according to their positions respective to protein coding genes [10]. Antisense lncRNAs are transcribed from the opposite strand of a protein-coding gene or a sense strand-derived RNA [19] whereas intronic lncRNAs are transcribed from intronic regions of either the sense or antisense strand [10]. The largest group, located between protein coding genes, are the intergenic lncRNAs (lincRNAs) [10]. Classes of lncRNAs that lack a poly (A) tail include: eRNAs (enhancer RNAs); sno-lncRNAs (snoRNA-related lncRNAs); circRNAs (circular RNAs); and ciRNAs (circular intronic RNAs) [39].

1.5 Mechanism of action of lncRNAs

Long non-coding RNAs (lncRNAs) are known to act via post transcriptional mechanisms by targeting splicing, stability, or translation of host mRNAs [4]. Long non-coding RNAs can also affect the expression of immune response genes through a variety of mechanisms [6]. It has been proposed that the antisense lncRNAs can be classified as mRNA-flanking lncRNA (mf-lncRNAs), despite their limited or no overlap with protein-coding genes [40]. This group of antisense lncRNAs include *THRIL* [15], *PACER* [41], *lincR-Ccr2-5OAS* [42], *lnc-IL7R* [43] and *IL1b-RBT46* [44], which have been reported to regulate the expression of their neighbouring protein-coding gene in *cis* [10]. They have also been reported to regulate the expression of many additional genes in *trans* [10]. Many of the reported immune-related lncRNAs, which are found in intergenic regions, regulate the immune response in *trans* [10].

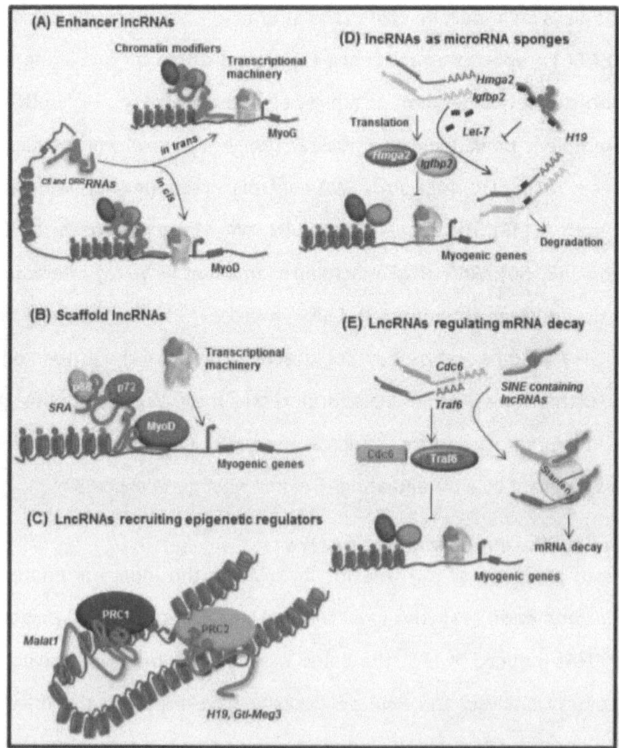

Figure 1.3 Different roles of long non-coding RNAs. Image sourced from Neguembor *et al*. [45].

One of the current mechanisms of most immune-related lncRNAs is believed to be through protein binding [10]. LncRNAs related to immune responses have been reported to be linked to members of the heterogeneous nuclear ribonucleoprotein (hnRNP) family [14, 15] and components of chromatin-modifying complexes including the polycomb repressor complex 2 [46], WD repeat domain 5, a core subunit of the MLL methyltrans-ferase complex [47], and the UTX/JMJD3 demethylases [48]. Though the mechanism is not clearly defined, it has been suspected that they might act as scaffolds to bring together proteins and/or target these to the DNA through base-pairing [28].

1.6 LncRNAs in host–pathogen interactions

Host lncRNAs produced by many pathogens are known to play significant roles in both the life cycle and/or interaction between intracellular pathogens and their host cells [10]. An example of a lncRNA that plays an important role in the interaction between HIV-1 and its host cells is *NEAT1* [49]. NEAT1 is reported to influence HIV-1 replication by regulating the nuclear-to-cytoplasmic export of Rev-dependent instability element containing HIV mRNA [49]. Another well-studied example is polyadenylated nuclear (*PAN*) *RNA* produced by Kaposi's sarcoma-associated herpesvirus (KSHV) [48]. *PAN RNA* controls viral gene expression and inhibits the host immune response [48]. The expression of *PAN RNA* is important in the switch from latent to lytic infection [48, 50]. *PAN RNA* mechanism involves physical interaction with LANA (latency associated nuclear antigen) [48]. LANA, a protein, is known to maintain latency by binding to the KSHV genome and modulating the dissociation of the protein once the virus is activated [48]. Furthermore, *PAN RNA* also suppresses the expression of host genes that are involved in the inflammatory and anti-viral response [48]. Overall, these studies suggest that lncRNAs play a significant role of regulating viral and host gene expression.

1.7 ncRNAs regulate the innate immune system

The first reported evidence of the role for lncRNAs in the innate immune response was reported by *Guttman et al.* [51] who used the intergenic deposition of epigenetic marks to identify 20 lincRNAs induced in LPS stimulated mouse bone marrow-derived dendritic cells (BMDCs). Microarray analysis and RNA sequencing have reported the differential lncRNA expression following activation by TLR agonists in monocytes, macrophages, dendritic cells, and fibroblasts, as well as following viral infection in mouse lungs [14, 15, 52-56]. There is a growing body of literature that reports on specific lncRNA involvement in host cell response to bacterial infections or stimulation with bacterial compounds. However, the functional role of lncRNAs in TB immunity is still very limited.

1.7.1 *LincRNA-Cox2* facilitates the induction and repression of gene expression in mouse macrophages

LincRNA-Cox2, located 50 kb downstream from the Cox2 gene, was first identified by [51]. This lincRNA was demonstrated to supress the expression of 787 genes in non- stimulated BMDMs and induce 713 genes following exposure to palmitoyl-3cysteinyl-seryl-4 (Pam3CSK4) [14]. *LincRNA-Cox2* and Ptgs2 were induced following exposure to LPS in BMDCs [14]. Gene Ontology analysis revealed that these differentially expressed genes were enhanced for genes involved in the immune response and included *CCL5* and *IL-6* [51]. The suppression of *lincRNA-Cox2* was facilitated through interaction with hnRNP-A/B and hnRNP-A2/B1 [14]. Sauvageau et al. [57] reported on the generation of a *lincRNA-Cox2* knockout mouse which provides an important resource for *in vivo* studies [57]. In their recent publication of the *lincRNA-Cox2* knockout mice they revealed that *lincRNA-Cox2* functions through an enhancer RNA mechanism to regulate Ptgs2 levels [58]. They also showed that *lincRNA-Cox2* has a *trans* regulatory role controlling many innate immune genes and the locus regulates the expression of local and distant genes [58] .

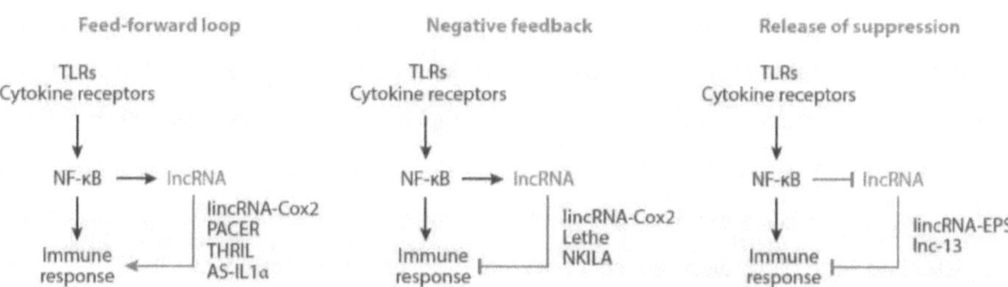

Figure 1.4 LncRNA-mediated regulatory circuits in inflammatory response in myeloid cells. Image sourced from Atianand et al. [12]

1.7.2 *THRIL* regulates TNF-α release and global gene expression in human monocytic THP-1 cells

Li *et al*. [15] showed that the expression of *THRIL* in THP- 1 cells is reduced post Pam3CSK4 stimulation [15]. Although this effect was indirect and dependent on autocrine/paracrine TNFα release, the knockdown of *THRIL* reduced the expression of 444 genes in unstimulated cells and downregulated the differential expression of 317 out of a total of 618 genes post Pam3CSK4 stimulation, these include many inflammatory genes such as IL6, CXCL8, CXCL10, CCL1, and CSF1 [15]. Similarly, with *lincRNA-Cox2*, *THRIL* was shown to interact with hnRNPL [15]. This resulted in the complex binding to the TNFα promoter and driving transcription in both control and Pam3CSK4-stimulated THP1 macrophages [15].

1.7.3 lincRNA-EPS regulates the expression of immune response genes in macrophages.

Using RNA sequencing, Atianand *et al*. [13] and colleagues identified lncRNAs that were downregulated in macrophages following LPS stimulation. One of the downregulated lncRNAs was *lincRNA-EPS* which was initially described as a regulator for erythrocyte differentiation [59]. lincRNA-*EPS* inhibits the expression of immune response genes (IRG) in both resting and

LPS stimulated macrophages [13]. Gain-of-function and rescue studies further confirmed lincRNA-EPS as a repressor of IRG expression [13]. The mechanism of *lincRNA-EPS* showed that it associates with chromatin and interacts with protein coding gene, hnRNPL, to inhibit the nucleosome positioning and repress IRGs [13]. *lincRNA-EPS*[-/-] mice had increased susceptibility to LPS challenge *in vivo* [13].

1.7.4 lncRNA Mirt2 is a negative regulator of inflammation

In this study Du *et al.* [16] and colleagues performed a microarray analysis in primary cultured peritoneal macrophages from C57BL/6 mice to identify lncRNAs that are involved in the innate immune response. *Mirt2* was among the highly induced lncRNAs by LPS stimulation [16]. They further show that *Mirt2* acts as a barrier to inhibit uncontrollable induction of inflammation, and is a potential regulator of macrophage polarization [16]. *Mirt2* was shown to associate with, and also reduce Lys63 (K63)-linked ubiquination of TRAF6 [16]. This association leads to the inhibition of NF-κB and MAPK pathways thus limiting the production of proinflammatory cytokines [16].

1.8 Functionally validated lncRNAs during Mtb infection

1.8.1 lncRNA-CD244 epigenetically controls CD8+ T-cell immune responses in tuberculosis infection.

CD4[+] T cells, CD8[+] T cells, and γδ T cells play important roles in establishing an adaptive immune response against Mtb infection [34, 60, 61]. CD244 is a costimulatory receptor important in the regulation of immune functions of Natural Killer (NK) cells [62]. It provides a negative signal that inhibits the activation signal provided by TCR engagement in CD8[+] T cells [63]. There is not much known on the molecular mechanism and consequence for CD244 regulation of T-cell effector functions during active TB infection. Wang *et al.* [64] examined whether CD244 signalling regulates T-cell effector function, how it affects homeostasis and host defence against Mtb infection [64]. Human lncRNA microarray and hierarchical clustering analyses were used to differentiate lncRNA expression in CD244[+] CD8[+] T cells and CD244[-] CD8[+] T cells [64].The microarray analysis identified highly expressed groups of lncRNAs differentially expressed in CD244[+] CD8[+] T cells [64]. They showed that *lncRNA-CD244* acts as an epigenetic regulator of IFNγ and TNF-α in production in CD8[+] T cells and impacts CD8[+] T-cell immunity against active Mtb infection [64].

1.8.2 The antituberculosis effect of lncRNA NEAT1

The differential expression and importance of *NEAT1* was analysed in active tuberculosis patients. PBMCs from patients with tuberculosis had increased expression of *NEAT1* [65]. *NEAT1* was markedly increased after Mtb infection in THP-1 macrophages [65], however silencing of *NEAT1* resulted in enhanced intracellular growth of Mtb and reduced IL-6 levels [65].

1.8.3 The role of lncRNA PCED1B-AS1

The authors examined the functional role of lncRNA *PCED1B-AS1* on macrophage apoptosis and autophagy [66]. LncRNA *PCED1B-AS1* expression was downregulated in patients with active tuberculosis [66]. Knockdown of lncRNA *PCED1B-AS1* reduced macrophage apoptosis and promoted autophagy [66]. It was also observed that lncRNA *PCED1B-AS1* serves as a sponge for miR-155 indicating that lncRNA *PCED1B-AS1* modulated macrophage apoptosis and autophagy by targeting miR-155 in active TB patients [66].

1.9 Functionally validated lncRNAs in *Mycobacterium bovis* BCG

1.9.1 LncRNA MEG3 eradicates mycobacteria in macrophages via autophagy

MEG3 was preselected due to its known role in immune related functions in cancer [67]. Human macrophages were stimulated with *Mycobacterium bovis* BCG and the expression of *MEG3* was analysed at early time points [68]. Using microarray analysis Pawar *et al.* [68] and colleagues showed the downregulation of *MEG3* after Mtb BCG infection. *MEG3* was linked to mTOR and PI3K-AKT signalling pathways therefore affecting the regulation of autophagy [68]. IFN-γ induced autophagy further reducing *MEG3* and knockdown of *MEG3* in macrophages resulted in autophagy and increased clearance of intracellular *M. bovis* BCG [68].

1.9.2 lincRNA-Cox2 induces intracellular mycobacterium killing in macrophages

LincRNA-Cox2 is upregulated by BCG infection in a time and MOI dependent manner [69]. Knockdown of *lincRNA-Cox2* reduces mycobacterium intracellular growth by induction of proinflammatory cytokines such as TNFα, IL-6, IL-12 [69]. The suppression of intracellular growth is also through inhibition of nitric oxide production [69]. Nitric oxide production is controlled through the NF-κB p50 and p60 subunits binding to the iNOS promoter [69].

1.10 Expression profiles of lncRNAs in immune cells infected with Mtb

Macrophages are well known in their important role in the controlling and clearing of *Mycobacterium tuberculosis* (Mtb) and also serve as host for Mtb [70]. Microarray analysis was used to investigate the expression profiles of lncRNAs and mRNAs in human macrophages infected with avirulent strains H37Rv and H37Ra [71]. The microarray analysis revealed differentially expressed lncRNAs [71]. Two lncRNAs, *MIR394HG V1* and *MIR394HG V2*, were identified as novel candidates for diagnostic markers for tuberculosis [71].

1.11 Differential expression of lncRNAs in serum, active TB vs healthy or latent individuals

Expression profiles of lncRNAs from PBMCs derived from healthy donors and donors with MDR-TB and drug sensitive TB (DS-TB) were analysed using the microarray assay [72]. A total of 1, 429 and 2, 040 lncRNAs were downregulated in MDR-TB and DS-TB groups, respectively [72]. The expression profile of long noncoding RNAS were investigated in serum using microarray analysis [73]. A total of 163 lncRNAs were upregulated and 348 were downregulated. Using Gene ontology (GO), Kyoto Encyclopedia of Genes and Genomes (KEGG) analyses they show that the functions of the differentially expressed lncRNAs were mainly associated with the regulation of alpha-beta T cell activation and T cell receptor signalling pathway [73]. Expression profiles of lncRNAs in CD4$^+$ T cells from latent and active TB donors were analysed using the microarray assay [74]. Compared to the healthy controls there was a total of 449 and 461 lncRNAs that were downregulated in LTBI, while 1, 113 and 1, 490 lncRNAs were downregulated in active TB group [74]

1.12 LncRNA interaction

1.12.1 LncRNAs and gene interaction

It has been reported that lncRNAs play a role in the epigenetic regulation of gene expression [75-77], and recent studies have proposed an integrated mechanism of action [78]. Protein complexes involved in chromosome modifications are recruited by lncRNAs directly or indirectly, which also results in epigenetic regulation [79]. Depending on the relative positioning between lncRNAs and their target genes, the mechanism by which lncRNAs regulate their target genes can be considered either *cis [80]* or *trans* [81]. LncRNAs that act in *cis* can regulate gene expression and/or chromatin state of neighbouring genes and those that act in *trans* are able to perform a variety of functions throughout the cell. In lncRNAs that have been reported to regulate target genes in *cis*, it has been shown that RNAs can form a nuclear complex that is linked to silenced genes [78]. Gene silencing is achieved through binding of lncRNAs to epigenetic modifiers [82]. An example is the *HOTAIR* lncRNA which inhibits gene expression in *trans* with Polycomb Repressive Complex (PRC) to regulate transcriptional inhibition of the HOXD locus [83].

1.12.2 lncRNAs and protein interaction

There is vast research showing how long non-coding RNAs function with their binding proteins [42]. Experimental methods such as mass spectrometry analysis followed by RNA immunoprecipitation have been used to identify lncRNA binding proteins [42]. A computational method called CatRAPID has been recently developed to predict RNA-protein interactions in the Xist network [84]. lncPro has been introduced as a new method to predict the interaction between lncRNAs and proteins [42]. Matrix multiplication is also used to score each RNA-protein pair as a measure of interaction within the pair [42]. This method distinguishes between interacting and non-interacting RNA-protein pair and predicts RNA-protein interactions within a given multiplex [42]. It was found that lncRNAs interacted with nuclear proteins and RNA-binding proteins when this method was applied on all human proteins [42].

1.12.3 lncRNAs and disease association

More and more studies are reporting that lncRNAs are implicated in a wide range of human diseases [41]. The dysregulation of lncRNAs has been reported to be the main cause of complex human disease processes [78]. *ANRIL* has been associated with coronary disease, type 2 diabetes and many other types of cancer [41]. *HOTAIR* expression is increased to over 200-fold in breast cancer metastases using qPCR [85]. *MALAT-1* is reported to be associated with metastases in NSCLC (non-small-cell lung carcinoma) patients by qPCR [86]. With regards to Alzheimeir's disease, *BCAE1-AS* was shown to regulate BACE1 and in driving pathology [87]. It is important to analyse the available lncRNA-disease associations and predict potential lncRNA-disease associations in human [41]. These analysis will help in understanding molecular mechanisms of human diseases and help identify biomarkers for disease diagnosis, treatment and prevention at lncRNA level [41].

1.13 lncRNA bioinformatics

1.13.1 LncRNAs secondary and tertiary structures

To understand the function of lncRNAs it is very important to study their structures and the interaction between their structure and sequence [78]. RNA has a unique ability to form secondary and tertiary folds [88]. The structural flexibility of RNA allows it to perform organizational, catalytic and regulatory functions [52]. Finding functional annotation of transcriptomes based on RNA structure has now become possible [89]. Due to the increasing number of lncRNAs discovered, powerful computational methods to predict RNA structure is necessary [78]. There have been a few structure prediction methods reported for non-coding RNAs [78].

1.13.2 Computational prediction of ncRNA secondary structure

The folding process of the majority of RNA molecules represents a transition between secondary and tertiary structure [90]. Finding the secondary fold of RNA is the initial step in finding out more about the functions of ncRNAs [88]. There have been a few methods that have been proposed to predict RNA secondary structure [78]. These methods are based on two different ideas namely the sequence alignments and the minimum free energy model [89]. MARNA, one of the methods, is a non-probabilistic approach which performs pairwise alignments considering the primary and tertiary structures [78]. The model folds sequences using free energy and then provides a structural alignment among a set of homologous sequences [78]. When the conservative sequence regions are visible, MARNA can predict the RNA secondary structure [78]. The total length of sequences analysed by this model cannot be longer than 10, 000 nucleotides [78]. Pfold is based on KH-99 algorithm which combines the evolutionary information and a probabilistic structure [78]. This model can accommodate a large number of sequences and able to predict a secondary structure when long sequences and large homologous sequences need to be analysed [78].

1.13.3 Computational prediction of ncRNA tertiary structure

The formation of specific tertiary structures is important for the functioning of ncRNAs in many biological processes [91]. RNAs can change their tertiary structures allowing them to interact with other RNAs, ligands and proteins or themselves [89]. 3dRNA is a method for rapid and automated building of RNA tertiary structure [78]. This method can find RNA tertiary structural templates from different RNA families [78]. 3dRNA is not limited to predicting tertiary structure and small RNA molecules and or those with simple topology [78]. It can predict for RNA molecules with a large size and complex topology [78].

1.14 The role of lincRNA-MIR99AHG in cancer

1.14.1 MIR99AHG and MIR100HG act as oncogenes in acute megakaryoblastic leukemia (AMKL)

MIR99AHG is transcribed as a polycistronic primary transcript that produces a spliced long intergenic noncoding RNA and three intronic miRNAs: *MIR99A*, *MIR125B2* and *LET7C* [29]. The *lincRNA-MIR99AHG* has a role in cell proliferation and differentiation [29]. However, the role of the lncRNA host genes in this ncRNA ensemble remained indefinable [29]. The function of *MIR99AHG* was characterized and a unique role of *MIR99AHG* was validated during hematopoiesis and the pathogenesis of acute megakaryoblastic leukemia (AMKL) [29]. *MIR99AHG* and *MIR100HG* are highly expressed in AMKL blasts [29]. The transcripts of these lncRNAs were mainly located in the nucleus and their expression correlated with the corresponding miRNA clusters. Knockdown of both these lncRNAs restrained leukemic growth of AMKL cell lines and primary patient samples [29]. Ectopic expression of *MIR99AHG* interfered with hematopoetic lineage decisions and increased the proliferation of immature erythroid progenitor cells [29].

1.15 Possible proximal genes adjacent to MIR99AHG gene

1.15.1 Cxadr

The coxsackie B virus and adenovirus receptor (CAR), located downstream of *MIR99AHG*, is a member of the immunoglobulin superfamily [92]. CAR is known to play a pivotal role for the entry of both coxsackie B viruses and adenoviruses in to host cells [93]. In addition to viral infection it also plays a role in maintenance of the junction adhesion complex in polarized epithelia and modulation of cellular growth properties [94]. In a publication by Giaginis *et al*. [93] and colleagues they revealed fort the first time the expression of CAR from patients with endometrial adenocarcinoma. CAR appeared to regulate the proliferation and characteristics of cancer cells thus its expression could be considered of possible clinical significance for gene therapy applications [93].

1.15.2 Usp25

Little is known about the molecular mechanism that controls downstream signalling from the IL-17R complex [95]. To understand the regulatory mechanism of this process, Zhong *et al.* [96] co-expressed various deubiquitinating enzymes with an NF-kB luciferase reporter construct and examined the reporter activity upon IL-17A stimulation. The assay revealed that the overexpression of the USP25, located upstream of *MIR99AHG*, significantly and specifically inhibited IL-17A- but not TNF-α-mediated NF-κB activation and the expression of inflammatory mediators [96]. USP25 binds to and deubiquitinates TRAF5 and TRAF6, thereby reducing NF-kB and MAPK signal transduction downstream of the IL-17R complex [96]. USP25-deficient mice displayed an enhanced IL-17A mediated inflammatory response when challenged with IL-17A *in vivo* or when subjected to IL-17A-related airway inflammation or experimental allergic encephalomyelitis (EAE) [96]. These findings demonstrate the physiological function of USP25 as a negative regulator of the IL-17R signal transduction pathway [96].

1.15.3 Bach1

In a study by [97], higher expression of miR-155 and miR-155* was observed in stimulated PBMCs of active tuberculosis patients as compared to unstimulated. Very recently, specific secretory *M. tuberculosis* antigen, ESAT-6 was also found to play a key role in miR-155 induction and its subsequent effects on Bach1 and SHIP1 repression [98]. It is known that Bach1 is a transcriptional repressor of haem oxygenase-1 and (HO-1) which is a documented activator of the *M. tuberculosis* dormancy, thereby favouring *M. tuberculosis* survival within mouse macrophages; whereas SHIP1 inhibits the activation of the serine/threonine kinase AKT (required for *M. tuberculosis* survival) [99]. Although Bach1 is located very far downstream of the *MIR99AHG* host gene, an interaction between this transcription factor and *MIR99AHG* was found in the human embryonic stem cell (ENCODE resource) [96]. Our group recently showed that Bach1 is a target for miR-143 and miR-365 which are both highly upregulated by Mtb infection [100].

1.15.4 Btg3

Btg3 is a member of the B-cell translocation gene (BTG) of ErbB2 gene family [101]. Btg3 is thought to be a negative regulator of the cell cycle and it has been shown that its anti-proliferative action through inhibition of the transcription factor, E2F1 [102]. It has also been shown that Btg3 is associated with the inhibition of Src tyrosine kinase [103]. Other studies have shown that Btg3 is a candidate tumor suppressor gene in human non-small lung cancer cell and oral squamous cell carcinomas [104]. In a study by Majid *et al.* [101], Btg3 gene was shown to be transcriptionally downregulated in renal cell carcinoma and that its mechanism of inactivation is through promoter hypermethylation.

1.16 Host-directed therapy as adjunct therapy

Host-directed therapies (HDT) are a promising and new therapeutic approach for treating tuberculosis. The use of HDTs is intended to increase the treatment of TB by immunomodulation and/or immune augmentation [105]. Therefore, HDTs are very important in achieving the 2035 WHO End TB goals [106]. Adjunctive HDT have the potential to shorten TB treatment duration, prevent antibiotic resistance and reduce lung injury by promoting autophagy, antimicrobial production and other macrophage effector mechanisms [3, 107]. So far, some HDTs have already been tested preclinical stages. Corticosteroids have been used as adjunctive therapy for many inflammatory and disease states [108, 109]. The rationale for using corticosteroids in active TB disease mechanistically involves modulation of inflammatory and apoptotic gene transcription pathways [110]. Corticosteroids as immunoadjuvants to standard TB treatments has proven to be useful in several studies including an HIV/TB coinfection framework [111-114]. Another promising candidate for host-adjunctive therapy for improving TB treatment is metformin. Metformin, an antidiabetic drug, has been shown to reduce the intracellular growth of Mtb in an AMPK dependent manner [115]. In two separate human cohorts, metformin has been shown to improve the control of Mtb and decreased disease severity [115]. The use of metformin in Mtb infected mice resulted in improved lung pathology, reduced chronic inflammation and enhanced the efficacy of conventional TB drugs [115]. Statins which are widely used to lower cholesterol levels, have broad anti-inflammatory and immunomodulatory activities [3, 116]. Statin treatment has shown potent adjunctive activity in a TB mouse model and mouse model of human-like necrotic TB lung granulomas [116]. Statin treatment and subsequent Mtb infection in mice resulted in increased host protection, reduced mycobacterial burden in the lungs, decreased dissemination and reduced pulmonary histopathology [117]. There are two clinical trials currently testing statins as adjunctive therapy for TB. Our research group is currently involved in a clinical trial that will test atorvastatin in reducing inflammation after TB treatment completion.

Many HDT approaches that have gained considerable research interest as adjunct to antibiotic-based anti-TB treatments include HDT targeting vitamin D pathway, HDT targeting autophagy, HDT targeting inflammatory response and HDT targeting cell-mediated immunity. A recent clinical study showed that co-treatment with phenylbutarate (PBA) and vitamin D_3 as an adjunct to standard chemotherapy reduces Mtb growth in MDMs and increases clinical recovery compared to the placebo group [118]. Carbamazepine drugs have been shown to stimulate autophagy through inositol triphosphate (IP_3) depletion and AMP- activated protein kinase activation and kill intracellular Mtb in macrophages [119]. In addition, carbamazepine treatment without ant-TB drugs reduced MDR-TB burden in lungs and spleen in mice [119]. Recently the first therapeutic RNA-based oligonucleotide was approved by the FDA and promises to be growing as many biopharmaceutical companies are developing RNA interference (RNAi)-based and RNA-based antisense oligonucleotide therapies [120]. The potential of using lncRNAs and miRNAs as adjunctive HDT is a topic that is gaining momentum especially in the context of infections and diseases. A handful miRNA-targeting drugs have entered into clinical trials targeting different diseases. [120]

1.17 Antisense oligonucleotide delivery
ASOs are oligonucleotides that function through the RNA interference (RNAi) pathway and inhibit mRNA translation [121, 122]. ASOs main aim is to inhibit a molecular target or RNA by induction of RNAse H endonuclease activity that binds the RNA-DNA heteroduplex with a substantial reduction of the target gene translation [123]. A different mechanism of action is through reduction of 5' cap formation, splice switching, and steric hindrance of ribosomal activity [121, 124, 125]. When developing ASOs it is very important to take into account off targets-effects and cytotoxicity [126]. The side effects of ASOs can be dependent on sequences and ASO backbone chemistry [126]. To avoid ASOs binding to non-targets, it is very important that the secondary and tertiary structures be taken into account to minimize wrong cleavage [127-129]. Most GapmeR ASOs are phosporothioated, meaning they are easily taken up thus limiting their bioavailability [130, 131]. Their chemical solubility does not affect the RNAse H activity or its solubility meaning they can easily be administered by different routes

(subcutaneous, intravenous, topical or rectal) [123]. Delivery of ASOs include naked delivery for localized treatments [132] , inhalation for pulmonary disease [133], transdermally for skin conditions [134] or in combination with other drugs [126].

1.18 FDA approved ASOs and ASOs in clinical trials
A few ASOs have been approved by the FDA. Formivirsen is an FDA approved compound administered intravenously to treat cytomegalovirus-induced retinitis [135]. Mipomersen is administered subcutaneously, for the treatment of homozygous familial hypercholesterolemia in the USA [136]. Eteplirsen, administered intrathecaly is used to treat Duchene muscular dystrophy [137]. Nursinersen, a recently approved FDA ASO used to treat spinal muscular atrophy, is administered intrathecaly [138]. Defibrotide is a compound administered intravenously, used to treat severe hepatic veno-occlusive disease [139].

There are a number of ASOs that are currently under trial. These compounds include NF-kB ASO has only been tested in murine models and despite encouraging results there is no available data in IBD patients [140]. Smad7 also known as mongersen ASO has been formulated to treat active Crohn's disease patients [141] and the phase III trial has been suspended due to reported lack of efficacy of mongersen. Nursinersen is also being clinically tested for amyotrophic lateral sclerosis (ALS), Huntington's disease and cerebellar ataxis, however delivery of ASOs remains a key challenge for translational success, especially for chronic diseases [137]

1.19 Research problem and focus
TB is known to hijack the host's immune response in the macrophages so it can persist and survive. Our research focus is to explore host factors such as lncRNAs and pathways that are overturned by Mtb to increase its persistence and survival within the host's macrophages. Host-factor targeting in macrophages is of primary concern because this is the area where Mtb initiates infection and develops persistence. This in turn will potentially affect the success of future target-based drugs directly. Our research group has already identified differentially expressed lncRNAs in M1 (IFNy) and M2 (IL-4/IL-13) activated macrophages [142]. This study will enable the identification of new potential targets and may offer interesting opportunities to produce innovative host-directed drug therapies against Mtb infection [3].

1.20 Aim

The aim of this study is to functionally validate lincRNA-MIR99AHG and validate its interacting partner in polarized and/or Mtb-infected macrophages using chemically engineered antisense oligonucleotides (GapmeRs).

1. 20.1 The objectives of the study:
1. Investigate the function of lincRNA-MIR99AHG and its target genes using chemically engineered antisense oligonucleotides (GapmeRs).

2. Predict lincRNA-MIR99AHG potential targets and interacting partners in polarized and Mtb-infected murine and human macrophages.

1.21 Hypothesis

Mtb hijacks host lincRNA-MIR99AHG to promote its intracellular survival in macrophages.

Chapter 2: Materials and Methods

2.1 Materials

All general reagents were purchased from either of the following suppliers: Merck Chemicals (Pty) Ltd.; Gibco Life Technologies; Corning, Invitrogen Life Technologies, Roche, and Sigma Aldrich. Molecular biology reagents were purchased from ThermoScientific, BD Bioeciences and Fermentas Life Sciences. See Appendix for reagents for all experiments.

2.2 Methods

2.2.1 Ethics Statement

The BALB/c mouse strain were bred and housed in specific pathogen-free conditions and all animal procedures were performed in compliance with the standards of practice for laboratory animal procedures set by the Animal Research Ethics Committee, Faculty of Health Sciences, University of Cape Town, Cape Town, South Africa (Ethics approval Ref 015/037). The recruitment of healthy volunteers for this study was approved by the Human Ethics Committee, Faculty of Health Sciences, University of Cape Town, Cape Town (HREC Ref Number: 635/2015). Inclusion criteria were as follows: age 18-50 years, both sexes, no history of TB, no contact with TB patients, HIV negative, sputum smear-negative, non-smokers, no chronic alcoholism, normal chest x-rays, no chronic disease, not receiving immunosuppressive therapy, IGRA negative and absence of other pulmonary diseases. The participants who did not meet the above criteria, did not consent to signing the information consent form or to undertaking an HIV test were excluded from this study.

2.2.2 Generation of Bone Marrow-Derived Macrophages (BMDMs)

Bone marrow-derived macrophages were generated from 8-11 weeks old male BALB/c mice. The mice were sacrificed using halothane and death was confirmed by cervical dislocation, and their femur bones were flushed using plain Dulbecco's modified Eagle's medium (DMEM) (Gibco, Invitrogen Corporation, Carlsbad, CA, USA) to collect (centrifugation: 1200 rpm; 4°C; 10 minutes) bone marrow cells. The cells were seeded in sterile 100 mm CORNING plates (14 x 10^6 cells/ml) and incubated (37°C; 5% CO_2; 70% RH) for 10 days in PLUTZNIK media (DMEM containing 10% Foetal Calf Serum, 5% horse serum, 2mM L-glutamine, 1mM Na-pyruvate, 0.1mM 2-beta-Mercaptoethanol, 30% L929 cell-conditioned medium, 100U/ml penicillin G, 100µg/ml streptomycin) to allow for their differentiation into BMDMs. On day 10, the adherent cells were lifted using 4mg/ml Lidocaine EDTA solution and gentle scrapping, thereafter, washed twice with DMEM (containing 10% FCS, 100U/ml penicillin G, 100 µg/ml streptomycin) to remove residual M-CSF (present in the L929 conditioned medium). The BMDMs were seeded at 2-3 x 10^6 cells/well, $5x10^5$cells/well and $1x10^5$ cells/well in 6, 24 and 96-well Nunc plates respectively and incubated (37°C; 5% CO_2; 70% RH) overnight before performing downstream experiments.

2.2.3 Generation of peripheral blood mononuclear cells (PBMCs) and monocyte-derived macrophages (MDMs)

PBMCs were isolated using Histopaque®-10771 (Sigma-Aldrich Biotechnology LP and Sigma-Aldrich Co., St Louis, MO) density gradient centrifugation. Blood was collected in VACUETTE® K3E blood collection tubes (Greiner Bio-one, GmbH, Germany), transferred to 50 ml Falcon tubes and diluted 1:2 with isotonic phosphate buffered saline (PBS) solution pH 7.4. 30 ml of diluted blood was transferred to 50 ml Leucosep™ 227290 tubes (Greiner Bio-one, GmbH, Germany) loaded beforehand with 15 ml Histopaque® solution as per the manufacturer instructions. The tubes were centrifuged at 1000 x g (2229 rpm) for 25 min (acceleration: 9; deceleration: 0) using an Eppendorf® 5810R centrifuge (A-4-81 Rotor, radius 18 cm). Plasma was discarded and buffy coat (lymphocytes / PBMCs) layer was harvested into a fresh 50 ml Falcon tube. The buffy coat was washed 3 times with 50 ml PBS solution pH 7.4 and spun at 250 x g for 10 min (acceleration 9, deceleration 5). PBMCs were re-suspended in 2 -5 ml complete growth medium (RPMI 1640 medium supplemented with 10% FCS, 2 mM L-glutamine and 1% penicillin G /streptomycin. All purchased from Life Technologies™, Carlsbad, CA, USA). PBMCs were plated at 1 x 10^5 cells per 96-well tissue culture plates (Corning Costar®, Cambridge, MA) in complete growth medium for downstream bacterial burden experiments.

For the generation of MDMs, PBMCs were plated in 6-/12-/96-well tissue culture plates (Corning Costar®, Cambridge, MA) at a density of 20/10/1 x 10^6 cells per well respectively and incubated (37°C; 5% CO_2; 70% RH) for 2 hours to allow monocytes to adhere. Non-adherent cells were discarded, and adherent monocytes were given a gentle wash with PBS then incubated in X-VIVO™ 15 serum free hematopoietic medium (supplemented with 1% penicillin G/streptomycin) for 7 days to allow for the differentiation of monocytes into MDMs.

X-VIVO™ 15 serum free hematopoietic medium was changed on day 4. On day 7, X-VIVO™ 15 was removed, MDMs washed once with PBS and complete growth medium added for downstream experiments. MDMs purity was assessed by fluorescence-activated cell sorting (FACS) analysis using a PE–labeled anti-CD11b; PerCP–labeled anti-HLA-DR; FITC–labeled anti-CD14 and APC–labeled anti-CD3 monoclonal antibodies (All purchased from BD Biosciences™ CA, USA). MDMs purity exceeded 95%.

2.2.4 Culture of RAW264.7 murine macrophage cell line

The murine macrophage cell line RAW264.7 were purchased from ATTC. The cells were cultured in an incubator (37°C; 5% CO_2; 70% RH) using DMEM medium supplemented with 10% Foetal Calf Serum, 4mM glutamine and penicillin/streptomycin (All purchased from Life Technologies™, Carlsbad, CA, USA).

2.2.5 Transfection of BMDMs and MDMs

MIR-99AHG MiRCURY LNA™ (Exiqon™/Qiagen, Germany) were diluted in Opti-Mem medium (Life Technologies™) and mixed in a 1:1 ratio with Lipofectamine 3000 (Life Technologies™). Cells were transfected with 25nM of the GapmeR: lipofectamine solution per well for 48 hours, depending on the downstream experiments.

2.2.6 Stimulation and *Mycobacterium tuberculosis* infection of BMDMs and MDMs

Macrophages were stimulated with recombinant mouse (100 units/ml) or recombinant human (10 ng/ml) IL-4, IL-13 or a combination of IL-4 and IL-13 (IL-4/13) (BD Bio-sciences). At 24 hours post-stimulation macrophages were infected with Mtb strain HN878 (clinical hypervirulent strain) at a multiplicity of infection (MOI) of 2 bacilli: 1 cell (2:1). After 4 hours, the supernatant was removed and fresh DMEM containing 10% FCS, 100U/ml penicillin G, 100µg/ml streptomycin, 10ug/ml Gentamicin with or without stimulants was added to remove extracellular bacteria. Two hours later, the medium was replaced with DMEM containing 10% FCS with or without stimulants. Included in an individual experiment, BMDMs were also infected with the laboratory strain Mtb H37Rv, HN37Ra and BCG for comparison of host response to the clinical hypervirulent Mtb strain HN878.

2.2.7 RNA Extraction

Cells were lysed in Qiazol (Qiagen, Germany) at different time point's post-transfection/-stimulation/-infection and lysates were stored at -80°C. Total RNA was isolated from the lysate using miRNeasy Mini kit (Qiagen, Germany) according to the manufacturer's instructions. RNA quantity and purity were measured using the ND-1000 NanoDrop spectrophotometer (ThermoScientific, DE, USA).

2.2.8 cDNA Synthesis and RT-qPCR

For protein coding gene expression analysis, 100 ng total RNA was reverse-transcribed into cDNA using Transcriptor First Strand cDNA Synthesis Kit (Roche, Germany) according to the manufacturer's instructions. Quantitative real-time PCR (RT-qPCR) was performed using LightCycler® 480 SYBR Green I Master (Roche, Germany) and gene-specific primers (IDT, CA, USA). Fold change in gene expression was calculated by the $\Delta\Delta Ct$ method and normalized to Hprt1 which was used as internal control. The non-stimulated 0 hour sample was set to 1. With regard to miRNAs, total RNA was diluted to 5ng/µl before cDNA was synthesised using miRCURY™ LNA MicroRNA PCR System First-Strand *cDNA Synthesis Kit* (Exiqon, Denmark) as per the manufacturer's instructions. qPCR was performed using miRCURY LNA™ Universal RT microRNA PCR New ExiLENT *SYBR® Green Master Mix* and microRNA *LNA*™ PCR *primer* sets for MIR99HG and HPRT as internal control (Exiqon, Denmark) in a Roche 480 Lightcycler (Roche, Germany). Fold expression was calculated using the $\Delta\Delta Ct$ method with non-stimulated 0hr sample set as 1 (calibrator). Protein coding gene, lncRNA and microRNA qPCR primer sequences and PCR run conditions are listed in supplementary table 1.

2.2.9 Bacterial Burden Determination

At 24- and 48-hours post-infection, supernatant was removed from Mtb-infected macrophages and stored at -80°C for analysis of cytokine production. Cells were lysed at 4- and 24-hours post infection in Triton X-100 and serial dilutions were plated on Middlebrook 7H10 agar plates and incubated for 15 days at 37°C in 5% CO_2. Colony forming Units (CFUs) were enumerated to determine bacterial burden.

2.2.10 Cytokine Production

Cytokine production was measured by enzyme-linked immunosorbent assay (ELISA) using ELISA development reagents (R&D systems, USA). Culture supernatants were diluted 2, 3 and 6 folds. Data was acquired using Versamax™ Tunable microplate reader with Softmax Pro v6.3. (Avantor®, US).

2.2.11 Griess reagent assay

Cultured supernatants were collected to measure protein levels of nitrite, which correlates to nitric oxide (NO) production, by Griess reagents prepared in the lab. Read out was acquired using Versama™ Tumble microplate reader with Softmax Pro v6.3 (Avantor®, US).

2.2.12 Arginase assay

Cells were lysed with Triton-X100 to measure Arginase activity with reagents prepared in the lab. Read out was acquired using Versama™ Tumble microplate reader with Softmax Pro v6.3 (Avantor®, US).

2.2.13 RNA pull-down assay

Biotin-labelled lncRNA-MIR99AHG were transcribed with biotin RNA Lbeling mix and T7 RNA polymerase (Promega), treated with RNase-free DNase I (Promega), and purified using RNeasy Mini Kit (Qiagen). Biotin-labeled lncRNA-MIR99AHG was mixed and incubated with nuclear extracts of BMDMs. Streptavidin-conjugated magnetic beads (Invitrogen) were added to each binding reaction and further incubated. Beads were washed thoroughly. Then the retrieved proteins were detected by Western blot.

Mass Spectrometry analysis a specific band present in the experimental lane will be extracted (corresponding region in the control lane will also be extracted). Gel pieces will be digested with trypsin and 10% of the peptides will be injected onto a C18 spray tip and eluted into the Orbitrap and analysed with a 35 minutes collision induced dissociated method.

2.2.14 RNA Immunoprecipitation (RIP)

HnRNPA2/B1 experiments were performed in nuclear extracts isolated from IL-4/IL-13 stimulated and/or Mtb infected BMDMs formaldehyde cross-linked conditions. Assays were performed as described in the Novex IP kit protocol (10007D) except that cells were crosslinked with 1% formaldehyde for 20 min. Nuclear extracts were precleared with protein G beads for 2 hours at 4°C and then incubated with control rabbit IgG or anti-hnRNPA2/B1 antibody (2μg per sample) for 2 hours at RT. RNA was collected from 800 μl of each sample using TRIzol and treated with DNase to remove contaminating DNA. MIR99AHG levels were analysed by TR-qPCR. The remaining 200 μl of each sample was collected, boiled for 10min and subjected to Western blot analysis.

2.2.15 Western blot

BMDMs were harvested and lysed in RIPA buffer supplemented with protease inhibitor (P-8340, Sigma-Aldrich, US). Protein concentrations in cell lysates were measured using Pierce™ BCA protein assay kit (23225, Thermo Fischer Scientific, US), and the same amount of protein was loaded and separated on a polyacrylamide gel. Proteins were transferred to a nitrocellulose membrane. Membranes were blocked with 5% BSA solution (prepared in TBST) for 2 hours and probed with primary antibodies overnight in dilution buffer (TBST supplements with 1% BSA). The antibodies used in western blots are: hnRNPA2/B1 (Santa cruz, sc-32316), hnRNPL (Abcam, ab6106), hnRNPK (Santa cruz, sc-28380), Cxadr (Santa cruz, sc-373791) and Gapdh (Santa Cruz, sc-365062). Membranes were probed with horseradish peroxidase-conjugated anti-mouse and anti-goat secondary antibodies (sc-2005 and sc-2020). Western blots were developed with LumiGlo Reserve™ chemiluminescent substrate kit (54-64-01, Sera care, Life Sciences, MA, US).

2.2.16 RNA sequencing and data analysis

WT BMDMs were transfected with LNA GapmeRs and infected with Mtb HN878 MOI 1:2 for 0, 4 and 24 hours. RNA seq libraries were prepared from total RNA and sequenced on Illumina HiSeq2000 as described by [143].

2.2.17 *In vivo* GapmeR challenge

Wildtype BALB/c mice were injected intraperitoneally with LNA GapmeR control (10mg/kg; Exiqon) or LNA GapmeR MIR99AHG (10mg/kg; Exiqon) for alternate days after 14 days of Mtb infection.

2.2.18 Histology

Lungs sections were collected from euthanized mice and placed in 4% formaldehyde solution. Embedded sections were then stained with heamatoxin and eosin (H&E), or chromotrope aniline blue (CAB). The percentage of free alveolar spaces was defined as the open spaces in whole lung sections in relation to the total lung tissue area. Both free spaces and tissue areas were measured using the area measurement tool by the Nikon microscope imaging software NIS-elements and the % of alveolar spaces was calculated in Excel. A blinded quantification was performed to measure the percentage of MPO, CAB, CD3, iNOS, and Caspase-3 using the Nikon microscope imaging software NIS-elements.

2.2.19 Flow cytometry

Assessment of BMDM activation into M1 or M2 state was measured by flow cytometry. For surface staining, cells were labelled with appropriate antibodies (MHC11 (M5/114.15.2), CD11b (M1/70), CD64 (PM8), CD86 (558703), CD80 (553769) CD206 (C068C2), Pdl.2 (TY25) purchased from BD Bioscience (Franklin Lakes, NJ, US) and eBioscience (San Diego, CA, US). After incubation, cells were resuspended in FACS buffer for acquisition. Acquisition was performed using BD LSRFortessa (BD Bioscience, NJ, US) and data were analysed using FlowJo software (Treestar, Ashland, OR, US).

2.2.20 Mtb infection and determination of burdens in mice

Anaesthetized mice were infected intranasally with 25 µl of viable HN878 Mtb bacilli into each nasal cavity with doses of 100 CFU/mouse for immune response analysis. Bacterial loads, histopathological and flow cytometry analyses in lungs of Mtb-infected mice were determined as previously described [144]. The lung weight index calculation was performed as a measure of inflammatory infiltration using: square root [(Lung weight in mg/Mouse weight in g) *10]/10. Briefly, aseptically harvested lungs and spleen were homogenized in 0.01% Tween-PBS and 10-fold dilutions were plated on 7H10 agar plates for the determinations of CFUs.

2.2.21 Cell viability and apoptosis

Assessment of apoptosis was analysed by flow cytometry using the FITC Annexin V Apoptosis Detection Kit II (BD Bioscience). After incubation, cells were resuspended in FACS buffer for acquisition. Acquisition was performed using BD LSRFortessa (BD Bioscience, NJ, US) and data were analysed using FlowJo software (Treestar, Ashland, OR, US). Cell viability was assessed usinf Cell Titer Blue (Promega, US). After incubation, data was analysed using Versama™ Tumble microplate reader with Softmax Pro v6.3 (Avantor®, US).

2.2.22 Statistical analysis

All data were analysed using GraphPad Prism v6.0, a Student's t-test (two-tailed with unequal variance) or unless otherwise stated in Figure legends. Means are shown as SEM., $*P < 0.05$, $**P < 0.01$, $***P < 0.001$ and $****P < 0.0001$, respectively.

Chapter 3: Mtb targets lincRNA-MIR99AHG for evasion in macrophages

3.1 Introduction

Tuberculosis (TB), caused by *Mycobacterium tuberculosis* (Mtb), is one of the leading infectious diseases in the world [1]. In 2018 it is estimated that TB caused more than 1.5 million deaths and globally 10 million people developed TB[1]. Mtb is primarily transmitted by the respiratory route, and while it is able to cause disease in most organs, the most occurring is pulmonary tuberculosis [8]. As more awareness is gained into host factors involved in pathogen killing, new insights that target the host-pathogen interaction have become significant especially as infectious pathogens affecting humans continue to infect and gain resistance from antimicrobials [3]. Mtb is able to utilize cellular host factors for its own survival and persistence [3]. By targeting and employing the host factors used by Mtb, this could lead to a reduction in pathology, mycobacterial burden and possible latency [3]. Immune cells are able to undergo changes in their transcriptional program in order to rapidly alter expression of genes which are important in host-defence [18]. The activation of the innate and adaptive immune cells is dependent on a coordinated set of transcriptional and post transcriptional events [18]. During these events many protein-coding genes are induced and repressed [18].

Long noncoding RNAs (lncRNAs) are a family of noncoding RNAs (ncRNAs) [22, 23] mainly characterised as >200 nucleotides [10]. lncRNAs are known to act via post transcriptional mechanisms targeting the splicing, stability, or translation of host mRNAs [38]. lncRNAs can act in *cis-* and *trans-* to regulate nearby genes or genes at other genomic locations [145]. Both *cis-* and *trans*-acting lncRNAS can activate or repress transcription through the recruitment of chromatin and modifiers [82, 146]. The function of lncRNAs in macrophage biology is recently emerging [12]. For example, *lincRNA-EPS* is an inhibitor of immune response gene (IRG) expression, acting as a regulatory checkpoint that is downregulated prior to inducible expression of IRGs [13]. Many other lncRNAs including *lincRNA-Cox2* [14], *THRIL* [15], *Mirt2* [16], *lnc13* [17] also regulate inflammatory genes in myeloid cells.

Recent studies have reported on the role of lncRNAs during Mtb infection. In other immune cells such as T cells, CD244 signalling in TB correlated with high levels of lncRNA-CD244 in the CD244+CD8+ T-cell sub-population and *lncRNA-CD244* acts as an epigenetic regulator of IFNγ and TNF-α production in CD8$^+$ T cells and impacts CD8$^+$ T-cell immunity against active Mtb infection [64]. *LncRNA-MEG3* was shown to eradicate mycobacteria in macrophages infected with *Mycobacterium bovis* (BCG) via autophagy by targeting the mTOR and PI3K-AKT signalling pathways [68]. A microarray study revealed expression profiles of lncRNAs in human macrophages infected with Mtb virulent H37Rv and avirulent H37Ra strains and two lncRNAs, *MIR3945HG V1* and *MIR3945HG V2* were identified as novel candidate diagnostic markers for tuberculosis [71]. However, our understanding of the functional role of lncRNAs in polarized macrophages and during Mtb infection with a hypervirulent strain and their clinical relevance is still limited.

In this study, we identify lincRNA-MIR99AHG which is abundantly expressed in IL-4/IL-13 polarized mouse and human macrophages and downregulated in PBMCs from active TB patients. LincRNA-MIR99AHG was shown to regulate inflammatory gene expression in macrophages stimulated with IL-4/IL-13 and infected with Mtb. We investigated the function and regulatory mechanism of lincRNA-MIR99AHG. Knockdown of lincRNA-MIR99AHG in Mtb-infected mice reduced the mycobacterial burden in lung and spleen. We found that lincRNA-MIR99AHG regulates the expression of its nearby gene Coxsackie virus and adenovirus receptor (Cxadr) by interaction with hnRNPB2/A1. We show that lincRNA-MIR99AHG is downregulated in active TB patients and Mtb infected human monocyte-derived macrophages (MDMs) *ex vivo*. We propose a model whereby IL-4/IL-13-induced lincRNA-MIR99AHG is a host-protective response following Mtb infection to inhibit Mtb intracellular survival and persistence in macrophages.

3.2 Results

3.2.1 MIR99AHG is induced by IL-4/IL-13 and repressed by Mtb HN878 infection

We previously utilized deep CAGE (Cap Analysis of Gene Expression) transcriptomics to define the transcriptome of M1 (IFN-γ) or M2 (IL-4, IL-13, IL-4/IL-13) activated bone-marrow-derived macrophages (BMDMs) [142] and during Mtb infection [147]. Using this approach (Figure 3.1A) we identified several differentially expressed lncRNAs with MIR99AHG being highly expressed in M2 (IL-4/IL-13) stimulated macrophages (Figure 3.1B). At 4 hours post stimulation, IL-4/IL-13 upregulated 150-fold the CAGE tags per million (TPM) expression of MIR99AGH when compared to the unstimulated macrophages. In contrast Mtb infection repressed MIR99AHG TPM expression in a time dependent manner (Figure 3.1C). The CAGE tags expression values of MIR99AHG was confirmed by RT-qPCR in cytokine stimulated and Mtb infected macrophages (Figure 3.1D-E). RT-qPCR also showed a slight induction of MIR99AHG by IFN-γ between 12 and 28 hours post stimulation (Figure 3.1D). This induction by IFN-γ was not as significant compared IL-4/IL-13 MIR99AHG induction in all three independent experiments performed. Altogether, these data show that MIR99AHG expression varies according to the macrophage polarization state, IL-4/IL-13 being the inducer and Mtb the repressor.

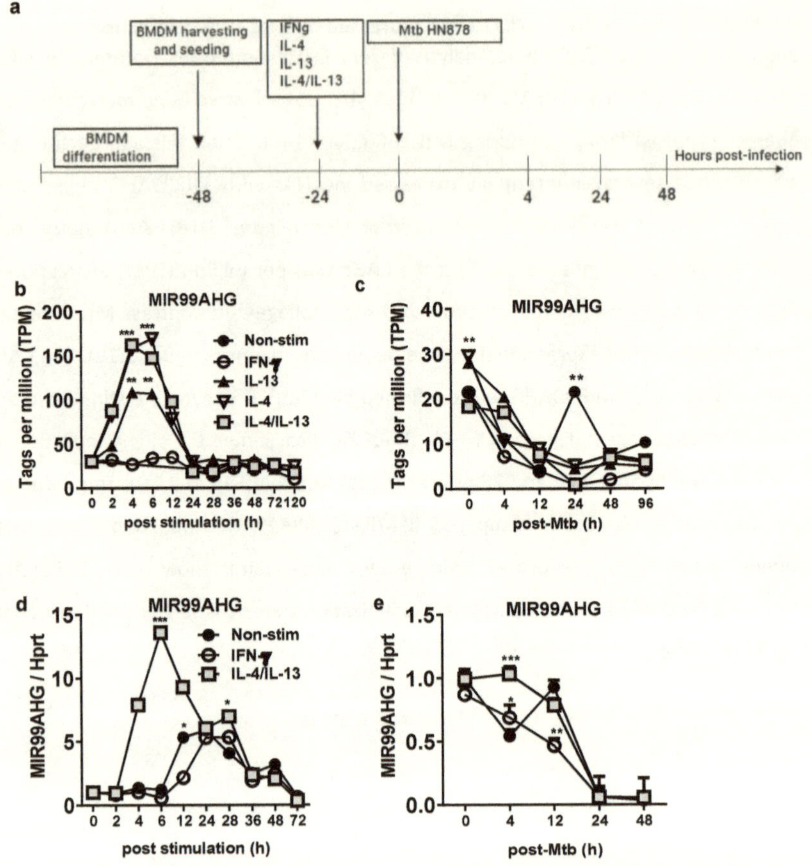

Figure 3.1 MIR99AHG is upregulated in M2 (IL-4/IL-13) activated macrophages and repressed in Mtb HN878-infected. (A-E) Bone marrow cells were differentiated for 10 days into BMDMs and stimulated with IFNγ or IL-4, IL-13, IL-4/IL-13. At 24 hours post-stimulation, BMDMs were infected with Mtb HN878 for 4, 24 and 48 hours. RNA was extracted from lysed cells at different time points post-stimulation and post-Mtb infection. **(A)** Timeline of mouse macrophage stimulation and Mtb HN878 infection.

(B, C) CAGE analysis of MIR99AHG kinetic expression in non-infected and Mtb-infected BMDMs following stimulation. Two-way ANOVA and Bonferroni post-hoc test was used to evaluate statistical significance. Three independent experiments were performed.

(D, E) RT-qPCR analysis of MIR99AHG kinetic expression in stimulated and Mtb-infected BMDMs. The fold change in gene expression was determined by RT-qPCR and was normalised to HPRT expression. Each data point represents arithmetic mean of triplicates ± SD. Three independent experiments were performed. Student's *t*-test was used to evaluate statistical significance, *P* values represented as, *$P<0.05$, ** $P<0.01$ and ***$P<0.001$.

3.2.2 Knockdown of MIR99AHG reduces intracellular Mtb growth and inflammatory cytokines

To examine the functional role of MIR99AHG in regulating intracellular growth of Mtb in macrophages, we performed lncRNA loss-of-function experiments using Locked Nucleic Acid (LNA) antisense oligonucleotides (ASOs) known as LNA GapmeRs. We first measured the knockdown efficiency in M2 (IL-4/IL-13) polarized macrophages and identified a 92% reduction of MIR99AHG expression at 4 hours post stimulation measured by RT-qPCR (Figure 3.2A). We also examined the knockdown efficiency at 48 hours post transfection (70%) (Figure S1A) and at 4 hours post Mtb infection (69%) (Figure S1B). LNA GapmeR treatment for control and MIR99AHG did not result in any toxicity during cytokine stimulation and Mtb infection as we identified stable cell viability measured by the cell titre blue assay (Figure 3.2B and Figure S1D and E).

To examine the functional role of MIR99AHG during Mtb infection, we inhibited MIR99AHG using LNA GapmeRs and analysed its effect on the intracellular growth of Mtb in macrophages by colony forming units (CFU) assays. Knockdown of MIR99AHG by LNA GapmeRs significantly reduced the intracellular Mtb growth in IL-4/IL-13 stimulated macrophages at 72 hours post Mtb infection (Figure 3.2C). Knockdown of MIR99AHG LNA GapmeRs led to an increased early apoptosis measured by AnnexinV+ and 7AAD- staining in IL-4/IL-13 stimulated BMDMs following Mtb infection, a possible mechanism of the reduced intracellular Mtb growth (Figure 3.2D). Nutlin is a known inducer of apoptosis. By RT-qPCR we confirmed apoptosis on BMDMs treated with nutlin and Mtb and there was an increased expression of Bax which is a pro-apoptotic marker and decreased Bcl2 expression an anti-apoptotic marker (Figure 3.2E and F).

To further characterize the functional role of MIR99AHG in cytokine production, we collected supernatant and RNA from LNA GapmeR transfected BMDMs and performed ELISA and RT-qPCR. Protein and mRNA levels of IL-6 (Figure 3.2G) and IL-1β (Figure 3.2H) were significantly reduced in LNA GapmeR treated for MIR99AHG when compared to the control in IL-4/IL-13 stimulated and Mtb-infected BMDMs. We measured nitrite production from BMDMs LAN GapmeR transfected, stimulated with IL-4/IL-13 and infected with Mtb. Knockdown of MIR99AHG by LNA GapmeRs reduced nitrite production compared to the control in IL-4/IL-13 stimulated and Mtb infected BMDMs (Figure 3.2I). Silencing of MIR99AHG by LNA GapmeRs in BMDMs stimulated with IL-4/IL-13 and infected with Mtb led to a decrease in CD86, a known marker for classically activated macrophages (Figure 3.2J). These data suggest that Mtb targets MIR99AHG to promote intracellular Mtb growth in macrophages regulates inflammatory host responses.

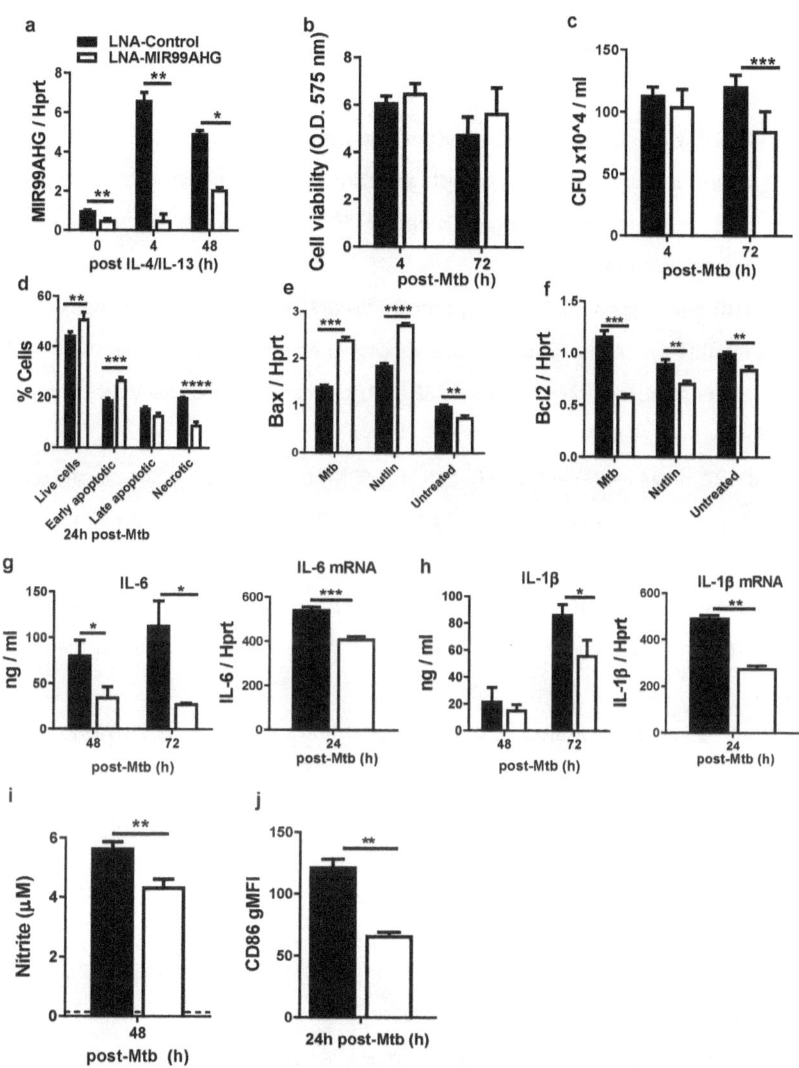

Figure 3.2 Knockdown of MIR99AHG reduces intracellular Mtb growth in macrophages. BMDMs were antisense oligonucleotides (ASOs) transfected with locked nucleic acid (LNA)-control and LNA-MIR99AHG, pre-stimulated with IL-4/IL-13 for 4 hours and infected with Mtb HN878. **(A)** Knockdown efficiency of LNA-GapmeRs analysed by RT-qPCR. Data representative of mean ± SD of triplicates. Three independent experiments were performed.

(B) Cell viability was measured in BMDMs at 4 and 72 hours post Mtb infection by Cell Titer Blue. Data representative of mean ± SD of triplicates. Three independent experiments were performed.

(C) MIR99AHG downregulation reduces mycobacterial growth in macrophages. BMDMs were lysed at 4 hours for uptake and 72h post-Mtb infection to measure mycobacterial growth by CFU counting. Data representative of mean ± SD of triplicates. Three independent experiments were performed.

(D) MIR99AHG downregulation favours apoptosis. BMDMs were stained with Annexin V+ and 7-AAD- to identify live, early apoptotic, late apoptotic, necrotic cells and measured by flow cytometry. Data representative of mean ± SD of triplicates. Two independent experiments were performed.

(E) Bax and Bcl2 mRNA expression by RT-qPCR in BMDMs treated with nutlin and infected with Mtb. Data representative of mean ± SD of triplicates. Three independent experiments were performed.

(G, H) Protein and mRNA cytokine levels of IL-6 and IL-1β measured by ELISA and RT-qPCR. Data representative of mean ± SD of quadruplets. Three independent experiments were performed.

(I, J) Nitrite production measured by Griess reagent and CD86 gMFI by flow cytometry 24 hours post Mtb infection. Data represented as mean ± SD of triplicates. Three independent experiments. *$P<0.05$, **$P<0.01$, ***$P<0.001$ and ****$P<0.0001$, Student's *t*-test.

3.2.3 *Cis*-acting MIR99AHG regulates the expression of nearby gene Cxadr

Cxadr is a protein coding gene located downstream of MIR99AHG whereas Usp25 is located upstream. We examined the *cis*-acting regulatory effects of the MIR99AHG on these two proximal protein-coding genes. Using LNA GapmeRs, we silenced MIR99AHG and measured Cxadr and Usp25 expression by RT-qPCR in IL-4/IL-13 stimulated and Mtb infected BMDMs (Figure 3.3A-B). At mRNA level , knockdown of MIR99AHG in IL-4/IL-13 + Mtb infected BMDMs significantly downregulated Cxadr expression, suggesting a positive *cis*-regulatory effect. In contrast Usp25 was upregulated by the silencing of MIR99AHG suggesting a negative *cis*-regulatory effect (Figure 3.3A-B). We employed Western blotting to further confirm the *cis*-regulatory effect on the cognate genes Cxadr which is located downstream of MIR99AHG

(Figure 3.3C). At 12 hours post infection, Mtb repressed Cxadr expression in a time dependent manner in IL-4/IL-13 stimulated macrophages (Figure 3.3D). In contrast, Mtb infection upregulated 350-fold the TPM expression of Usp25 in IL-4/IL-13 stimulated macrophages at 4 hours post Mtb infection (Figure 3.3E).

To assess the impact of MIR99AHG silencing on host immune response genes in macrophages, we performed RNA-seq in MIR99AHG knockdown BMDMs infected with Mtb for 4 and 24 hours. The silencing of MIR99AHG altered the expression of 441 and 679 genes at 4 and 24 hours post Mtb infection, respectively (P < 0.05) $\log_2$-fold change > 2. We identified 35 genes that were commonly upregulated and 26 genes that were commonly downregulated by MIR99AHG knockdown (Figure 3.3F). Most genes were genes were upregulated at 24 hours post Mtb infection. The upregulated genes were significantly enriched in terms related to regulation of inflammatory responses, response to bacteria, apoptotic cell death, and regulation of Erk1/2 cascade and activation of innate immune response (Figure 3.3G).

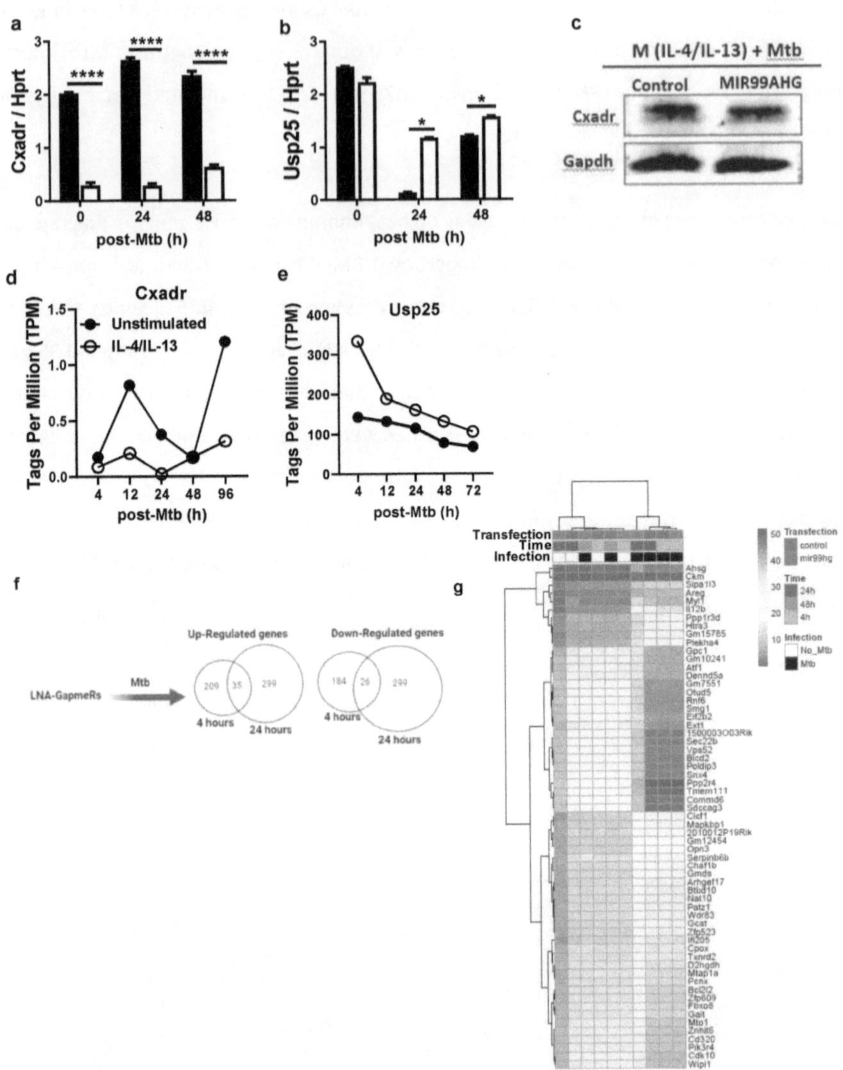

Figure 3.3 *Cis*-acting MIR99AHG regulates expression of nearby gene, Cxadr. (A-C) BMDMs were antisense oligonucleotides (ASOs) transfected with locked nucleic acid (LNA)-control and LNA-MIR99AHG, pre-stimulated with IL-4/IL-13 for 4 hours and infected with Mtb HN878. **(A, B)** mRNA expression of mouse Cxadr and Usp25 analysed by RT-qPCR. Data representative of mean ± SD of triplicates. Three independent experiments were performed.

(C) Protein expression of mouse Cxadr and Usp25 analysed by western blot. Three independent experiments were performed.

(D-E) CAGE analysis of Cxadr and Usp25 kinetic expression in BDMDs pre-stimulated with IL-4/IL-13 and later Mtb infected. Data representative of mean ± SD of triplicates. Three independent experiments were performed.

(F) Venn diagrams displaying the differentially expressed genes from LNA GapmeR transfected and Mtb infected BMDMs for 4 and 24 hours.

(G) Heatmap of representative genes commonly upregulated and downregulated in MIR99AHG knockdown BMDMs between 4 and 24 of hours. Data are represented as mean ± SD of triplicates. Data shown is representative of three independent experiments. *P<0.05, and ****P<0.0001, Student's *t*-test.

3.2.4 *In vivo* treatment with LNA GapmeRs for MIR99AHG reduced mycobacterial burden in mice

To compare the expression of MIR99AHG *in vivo*, we examined whole lung from Mtb infected mice or naïve lungs by RT-qPCR. MIR99AHG was downregulated in mice infected with Mtb at 11 and 21 days post infection (Figure 3.4A). To confirm whether MIR99AHG suppression is virulence dependent, we infected BMDMs with different Mtb strains and examined the expression of MIR99AHG post Mtb infection (Figure S3A). *Mycobacterium bovis* (BCG) induced MIR99AHG expression while the virulent strains H37Rv and hypervirulent strain HN878 inhibited MIR99AHG expression (Figure S2A). We also observed a similar suppression of MIR99AHG from whole lung infected with the Mtb clinical isolate CDC1551 and the virulent N0072 strain (Figure S2B). Targeting of noncoding RNAs to promote host innate defence is a promising strategy in the development of novel therapeutic interventions against TB [148, 149]. To investigate whether the beneficial effects of MIR99AHG suppression could be translated into a host-directed therapy (HDT), we used Antisense LNA GapmeRs to inhibit MIR99AHG in a mouse Mtb infection model and tested its prophylactic efficacy. Mtb downregulates MIR99AHG, hence we employed a prophylactic treatment before Mtb infection to inhibit MIR99AHG. First, the mice were subcutaneously treated with LNA GapmeR for MIR99AHG or NC (negative control) at 10 mg/kg for alternate days up to day 14. Mice were then infected with the hypervirulent Mtb HN878 strain (100 CFU/mouse) intranasally for 21 days. There was no difference in the Mtb uptake into lungs measured by colony forming units (CFU) assay at day 1 post infection between both treated groups, excluding possible role for different Mtb inoculation variable on the subsequent mycobacterial burden (Figure 3.4B). RT-qPCR results showed LNA-MIR99AHG GapmeR prophylaxis treatment drastically supressed MIR99AHG expression in lung tissues with a knockdown (KD) efficiency of 73% (Figure 3.4C). MIR99AHG KD mice showed significant reduced mycobacterial load in the lungs and in the spleen when compared to LNA GapmeR treated mice control mice (Figure 3.4D-E).

At 3 weeks post infection there was no difference in lung weight index, and total lung cells between the control mice and MIR99AHG KD mice (Figure 3.4F-G). Lung inflammation was quantified by measuring alveolar spaces which were significantly increased in MIR99AHG KD mice compared to the control mice, indicative of reduced pulmonary lesions in MR99HAG KD mice (Figure 3.4H). Neutrophil influx into lungs was also reduced in MIR99AHG KD mice, quantified by tissue-damaging factor myeloperoxidase (MPO) staining (Figure 3.4I). T cell recruitment measured by CD3 staining was significantly reduced (Figure 3.4J). There was no significant different between the two groups in CAB (Chromotope Aniline Blue) staining indicating that that fibrotic tissues were similar between both groups (Figure 3.4K). Caspase-3, a marker for apoptosis was increased in MIR99AHG KD mice compared to the control group (Figure 3.4L). iNOS, the enzyme responsible for producing the anti-mycobacterial effector molecule nitric oxide, was significantly reduced in MIR99AHG KD mice compared to the control group (Figure 3.4M, N). Also, at 3 weeks post infection MIR99AHG KD mice resulted in significantly reduced histopathology (H&E) in lungs compared to the control mice (Figure 3.4N). Taken together, these results suggest in that MIR99AHG during Mtb infection contributes to increased histopathology due to increased pulmonary inflammation.

To confirm if other infectious pathogens had a similar effect on the expression of MIR99AHG, whole spleen and lung of mice infected *with Listeria monocytogenes* showed downregulation of MIR99AHG (Figure S2C-D). This downregulation was also observed in BMDMs stimulated and infected with *Leishmania mexicana* (Figure S2E) suggesting that MIR99AHG is also downregulated by other intracellular pathogens.

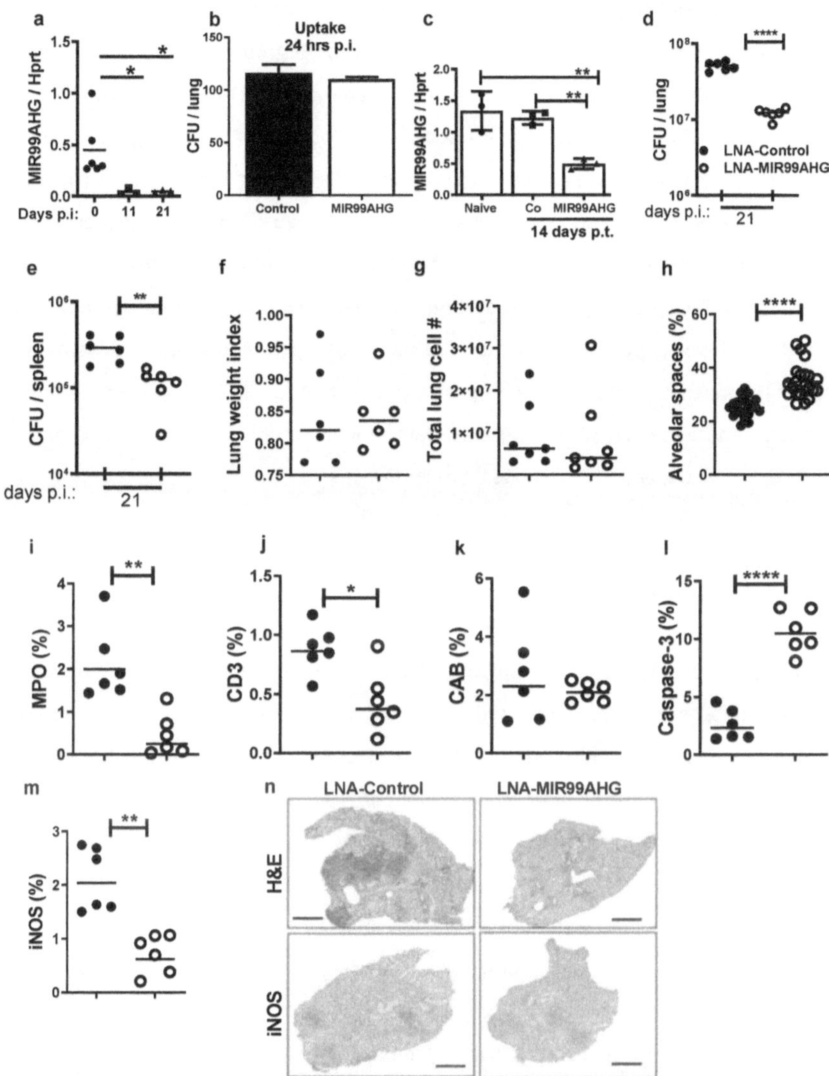

Figure 3.4 Inhibition of MIR99AHG *in vivo* impedes intracellular survival of Mtb in mice. (A)
RT-qPCR analysis of MIR99AHG expression on whole lung from wild-type (WT) mice infected
with Mtb HN878 (100 CFU/mouse) for 11 and 21 days. BALB/c mice (n=6/mice/group) were
antisense oligonucleotide (ASO) treated with 10 mg/kg locked nucleic acid (LNA)-control and
LNA-MIR99AHG. (A) Knockdown efficiency (73%) of MIR99AHG at 14 days post ASO

treatment, analysed by RT-qPCR. (B) Mtb-infected mice were sacrificed at 24 hours post infection to determine the CFU lung uptake (n = 3 mice/per group). **(C)** Knockdown efficiency (73%) of MIR99AHG at 14 days post ASO treatment, analysed by RT-qPCR. **(D-E)** Mycobacterial burden of Mtb HN878-infected mice are shown with indicated CFU in lung and spleen at 3 weeks post infection. **(F)** Lung weight index and **(G)** Total lung cell numbers. **(H)** Alveolar spaces at 3 weeks post infection were quantified from 4 deep cut H&E lung sections per mice (30 μm apart). **(I-M)** The percentage of positive MPO, CD3, CAB (Chromotrope Aniline Blue), Caspase-3 and iNOS staining per lung section was quantified from 1-2 deep cut lung sections per mice at 3 weeks post Mtb infection (30 μm apart). **(N)** Representative histopathology sections (x2 magnification) at 3 weeks post Mtb infection for H&E (scale bar=1000 μm). All error bars denote mean ± SD of triplicates. Data shown is representative of one experiment. *P < 0.05, **P<0.01, and ***P < 0.0001; Student's t-test

3.2.5 MIR99AHG leads to TB disease progression by inducing pro-inflammatory responses in the lung macrophages

To better define cellular infiltration in the lungs, cell populations were analysed by flow cytometry, at 3 weeks post-infection with 100 CFU/mouse of Mtb HN878. There were no significant differences in number and percentages of alveolar macrophages, interstitial recruiting macrophages and monocyte-derived macrophages between the MIR99AHG KD mice and the control mice (Figure 3.5A, Figure S3A). Percentages of DCs were significantly higher and neutrophils significantly lower in MIR99AHG KD mice compared to the control (Figure 3.5B-C), however there was no significant differences in cell numbers (Figure S3B-C). T lymphocyte population in the lungs were not affected by the knockdown of MIR99AHG except for increased percentage of CD4$^+$ T$_{effector}$ cells (Figure 3.5D-E, Figure S3D-E).

FACS sorting of neutrophils, alveolar macrophages, MoDCs and interstitial recruited macrophages population confirmed the silencing of MIR99AHG, with the control group still producing a significant amount of MIR99AHG (Figure 3.5F). Notably, alveolar and recruited interstitial macrophages from Mtb-infected MIR99AHG KD mice resulted in reduced levels of pro-inflammatory cytokines, such as *il1b* and *il6* compared to control cells (Figure 3.5G-H). Anti-inflammatory cytokines *il10* and *tgfb* were significantly reduced in alveolar and recruited interstitial macrophages and monocyte derived macrophages (Figure 3.5I-J). In addition, *Nos2* was significantly reduced in alveolar and recruited interstitial macrophages from Mtb-infected MIR99AHG knockdown mice (Figure 3.5K). Similarly, M2 markers Arg1, Ym1 and Mrc1 were significantly downregulated in alveolar, recruited interstitial macrophages and monocyte derived macrophages (Figure 3.5L-N). These results indicate that MIR99AHG is involved in early inflammatory responses suggesting that alveolar, recruiting interstitial and monocyte derived macrophages post Mtb-infection increase TB disease progression.

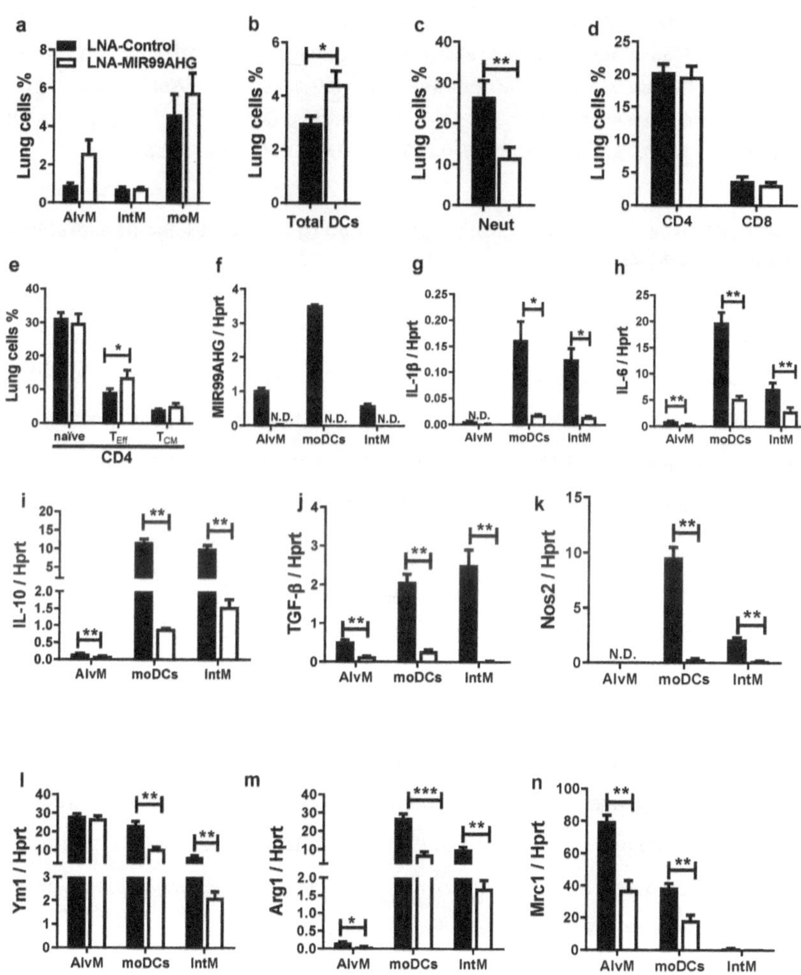

3.2.6 MIR99AHG is repressed in macrophages exposed to TLR ligands and its expression is dependent on IL-4Rα signalling

We employed RT-qPCR to examine the kinetics of MIR99AHG expression in BMDMs exposed to TLR ligands including LPS (TLR 4) and Pam3CSK4 (TLR2/1). The response of MIR99AHG was downregulated in BMDMs (Figure 3.6A) exposed to LPS and Pam3CSK4. Selective pharmacological inhibitors for NF-κB (Bay11-7084), Erk1/2 (FR180204, extracellular signal-regulated kinase) and p38 (SB203580) were used to assess the functional consequences of inhibition of these pathways on MIR99AHG expression. Pre-treatment with Bay11-7084 and SB203580 upregulated MIR99AHG expression in LPS stimulated macrophages (Figure 3.6B-C). In addition, the selective Erk1/2 inhibitor FR180204 exerted inhibitory effects of MIR99AHG expression on Mtb infected BMDMs (Figure 3.6D). Induction of IL-6 and IL-1β was impaired in BMDMs pre-treated with FR180204 post Mtb infection (Figure 3.6E-F).

Next, we sought to measure the expression MIR99AHG in MYD88$^{-/-}$ and IL-4Rα$^{-/-}$ mice. The TLR4 signalling is dependent on MYD88 and TRIFF [150], while IL-4 signals through two different receptor complexes, IL-4Rα or and IL-13Rα1 [151]. Since MIR99AHG is upregulated by IL-4/IL-13, we examined the expression of MIR99AHG in IL-4Rα$^{-/-}$ BMDMs and we observed a down regulation of MIR99AHG compared to the wild type in IL-4/IL-13 stimulated BMDMs (Figure 3.6G). In contrast, MIR99AHG expression was upregulated in IL-4Rα$^{-/-}$ BMDMs infected with Mtb compared to WT BMDMs (Figure 3.6H). MIR99AHG expression was downregulated in MYD88$^{-/-}$ BMDMs post LPS stimulation (Figure 3.6I). This suggests that MYD88 is not involved in the control of MIR99AHG expression in LPS induced BMDMs. Collectively, these results indicate that MIR99AHG levels in macrophages are dynamically regulated in response to microbial and inflammatory triggers.

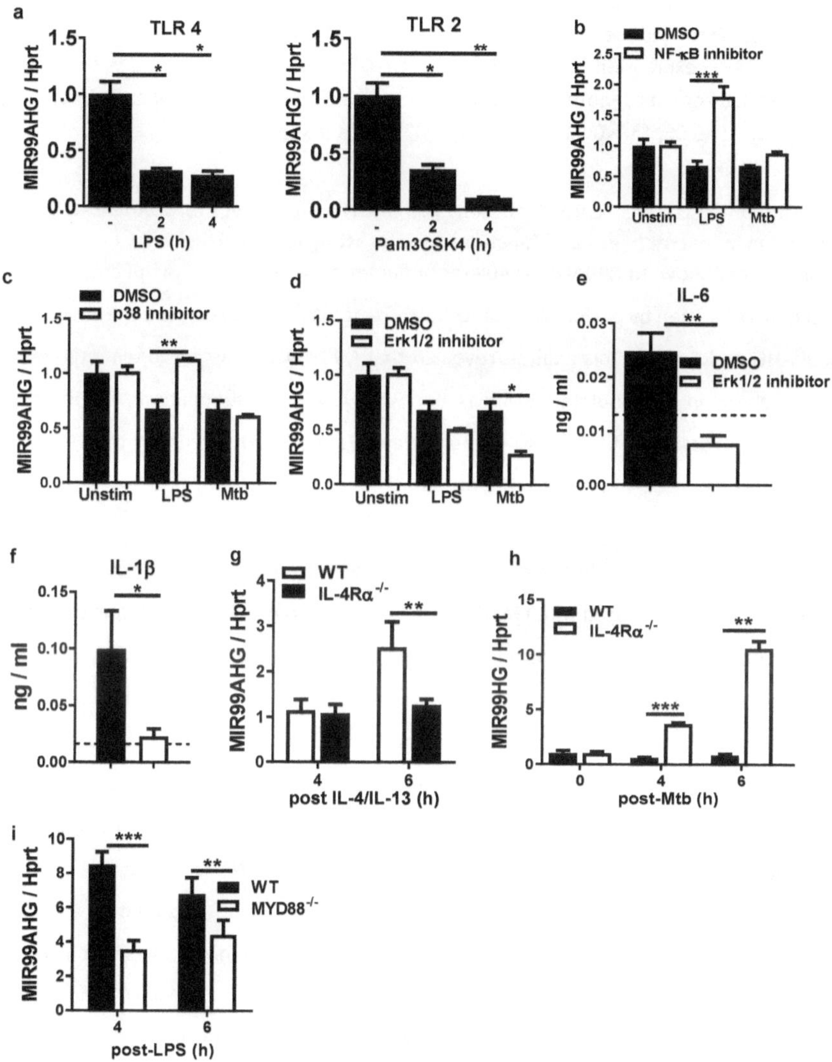

Figure 3.6 MIR99AHG is repressed in macrophages exposed to TLR ligands. (A) RT-qPCR of MIR99AHG mRNA expression on BMDMs exposed to TLR-4 agonist (LPS, 100 ng/ml), TLR-2 agonist (Pam3Csk4, 100 ng/ml). **(B-D)** RT-qPCR of MIR99AHG mRNA expression on BMDMs

44

were pre-treated for 1 hour with selective pharmacological inhibitors for NF-κB (Bay11-7084, 10 μM), p38 (SB203580, 5 μM) and Erk1/2 (FR180204, 10 μM), then activated by LPS stimulation (100 ng/ml) for 24h or infected with Mtb HN878 (MOI 1:2) for 24h. Data representative of mean ± SD of triplicates. Three independent experiments were performed. **(E, F)** IL-6 and IL-1β protein production measured by ELISA. Data representative of mean ± SD of triplicates. Three independent experiments were performed.
(G-I) MIR99AHG expression from IL-4Rα$^{-/-}$ and MYD88$^{-/-}$ BMDMs stimulated with IL-4/IL-13, LPS and Mtb. Error bars denote mean ± SD of triplicates. Three independent experiments were performed. *$P<0.05$, **$P<0.01$ and ***$P<0.001$, Student's t-test.

3.2.7 MIR99AHG is translocated from the cytoplasm to the nucleus following IL-4/IL-13 stimulation in macrophages and functions by interacting with hnRNPA2/B1

To understand how MIR99AHG regulates inflammatory responses in macrophages, we examined its location by performing sub-cellular fractionation and analysed the expression of MIR99AHG by RT-qPCR. This analysis revealed that MIR99AHG was predominantly found in the cytoplasm in unstimulated BMDMs but with IL-4/IL-13 stimulation we observed a significant expression of MIR99AHG in the nucleus (Figure 3.7A) suggesting that MIR99AHG may exert its biological functions in the nucleus.

To identify MIR99AHG binding proteins, we performed RNA pulldown assay by incubating *in vitro* transcribed biontylated MIR99AHG and its antisense control RNA with nuclear extracts from IL-4/IL-13 stimulated and Mtb infected BMDMs. The associated proteins were pulled down and analysed by mass spectrometry. We identified the 6 most enriched MIR99AHG-binding proteins based on the number of peptides specifically associated with MIR99AHG (Figure 3.7B). Among the 6 genes examined, hnRNPA2/B1 had the highest number of peptides associated with MIR99AHG (Figure 3.7B). To confirm hnRNPA2/B1-MIR99AHG interaction we performed RNA immunoprecipitation (RIP) of endogenous hnRNPA2/B1 nuclear extracts of IL-4/IL-13 stimulated and Mtb infected BMDMs followed by RT-qPCR and western blot (Figure 3.7C-D). Though we show MIR99AHG-hnRNPA2/B1 interaction, more studies that investigate the functional consequences of the inhibition of hnRNPA2/B1 on MIR99AHG and its target genes still need to be explored to fully substantiate this interaction. Altogether, these data show that MIR99AHG is translocated to the nucleus upon IL-4/IL-13 stimulation and interacts with hnRNPA2/B1.

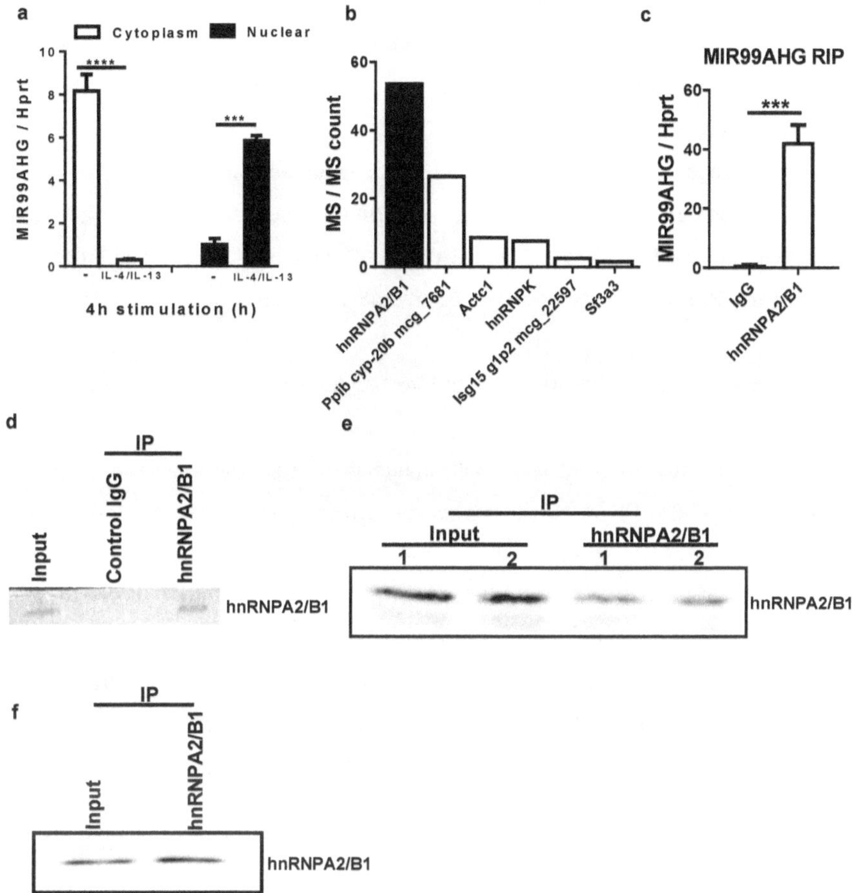

Figure 3.7 MIR99AHG is localized in the nucleus in IL-4/IL-13 stimulated macrophages and functions by interacting with hnRNPA2/B1. (A) RT-qPCR analysis of RNAs purified from nuclear and cytoplasm compartments in BMDMs stimulated with IL-4/IL-13 for 4h. Data representative of mean ± SD of triplicates. Three independent experiments were performed. **(B)** Candidate MIR99AHG-binding proteins identified by mass spectrometry. Data shown Srepresentative of one experiment.

(C) RT-qPCR analysis of MIR99AHG in anti-hnRNPA2/B1 antibody or control IgG immunoprecipitates from nuclear lysates of LNA-Control or LNA-MIR99AHG knockdown macrophages stimulated with IL-4/IL-13 and infected with Mtb. Error bars denote mean ± SD of triplicates. Data shown are representative of one experiment.

(D) Western blot analysis of hnRNPA2/B1 in Input, anti-hnRNPA2/B1 antibody and control IgG immunoprecipitates from nuclear lysates of LNA-Control or LNA-MIR99AHG knockdown macrophages stimulated with IL-4/IL-13 and infected with Mtb. Data shown are representative of one experiment.

(E, F) Western blot analysis of hnRNPA2/B1 in Input and anti-hnRNPA2/B1 antibody immunoprecipitates from nuclear lysates of LNA-MIR99AHG knockdown macrophages stimulated with IL-4/IL-13 and infected with Mtb. Data shown are representative of two experiments. ***$P < 0.001$ and ****$P < 0.0001$, Student's *t*-test.

3.2.8 Suppression of MIR99AHG in Mtb-infected human macrophages and active TB patients

To confirm the mouse macrophages results in human macrophages, we have examined the expression of MIR99AHG in human monocyte-derived macrophages (MDMs). Similar to BMDMs, MIR99AHG was upregulated by IL-4/IL-13 stimulation and downregulated by Mtb HN878 infection (Figure 3.8A-B). We employed RT-qPCR to examine the kinetics of MIR99AHG expression on LNA GapmeR transfected human MDMs exposed to IL-4/IL-13 and Mtb infection. The expression of MIR99AHG was downregulated after stimulation and Mtb infection (Figure S4A-B). Cell viability was confirmed on human MDMs by CellTitre-blue (Figure S4D-F). Knockdown of MIR99AHG with LNA GapmeRs reduced Mtb intracellular growth in MDMs (Figure 3.8C). mRNA levels of Bax were increased in nutlin treated and Mtb infected macrophages treated with LNA GapmeR for MIR99AHG (Figure S4G-H). Knockdown of MIR99AHG with LNA GapmeRs in MDMs stimulated with IL-4/IL-13 followed by Mtb infection reduced IL-6 protein levels (Figure 3.8D).

Next, we examined MIR99AHG expression in MDMs from healthy donors infected with Mtb HN878. There was a suppression of MIR99AHG post Mtb infection in a time dependent manner (Figure 3.8E). Human CXADR was also downregulated in a time dependent manner post Mtb infection (Figure 3.8F). Finally, we re-stimulated PBMCs from active and healthy TB patients with IL-4/IL-13 and heat killed (HK) Mtb. MIR99AHG expression is reduced in active TB patients compared to healthy patients (Figure 3.8G). Taken together these results demonstrate that MIR99AHG is suppressed in Mtb-infected human macrophages and in TB patients.

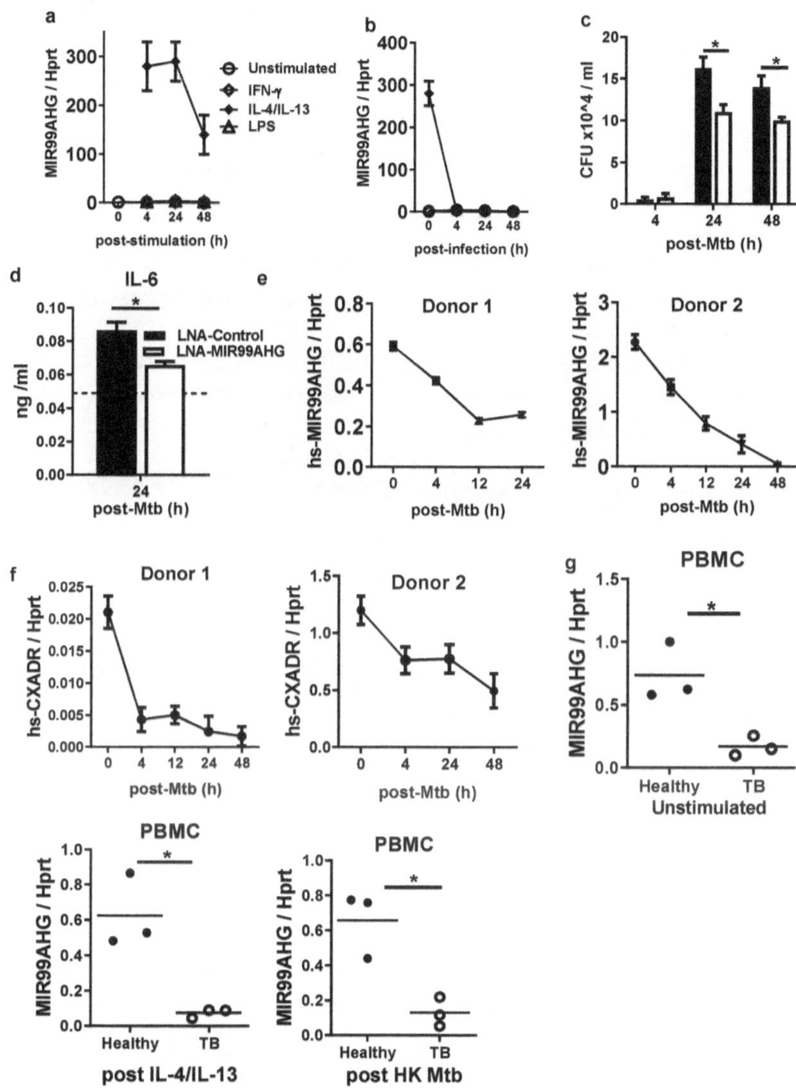

Figure 3.8 Suppression of MIR99AHG in Mtb-infected human macrophages and active TB patients. (A) RT-qPCR analysis of MIR99AHG kinetic expression in stimulated and **(B)** Mtb-infected MDMs. Data representative of mean ± SD of triplicates. Data representative of one experiment.

(C) MDMs were LNA GapmeR transfected with control and MIR99AHG, pre-stimulated with IL-4/IL-13 for 4 hours and infected with Mtb HN878. Cells were lysed at 4h for uptake and 24 and 48h post-Mtb infection to measure bacterial growth by CFU counting. Data representative of mean ± SD of triplicates. Three independent experiments were performed.

(D) IL-6 production on MDMs pre-stimulated with IL-4/IL-13 and infected with Mtb HN878 measured by ELISA. Data representative of mean ± SD of triplicates. Three independent experiments were performed.

(E) RT-qPCR analysis of human MIR99AHG expression on MDMs from healthy donors infected with Mtb HN878. Data representative of mean ± SD of triplicates. Three independent experiments were performed.

(F) RT-qPCR analysis of human CXADR expression on MDMs from healthy donors infected with Mtb (HN878) *ex vivo*. Data representative of mean ± SD of triplicates. Three independent experiments were performed.

(G) Re-stimulated PBMCs from healthy and active TB patients analysed by RT-qPCR. Error bars denote mean ± SD of triplicates. Data shown are representative of one experiment. P values represented as, *P<0.05, Student's *t*-test.

3.3 Discussion

Mtb is an intracellular pathogen that can evade lysosomal degradation and establish persistent infections. Host-directed drug therapies (HDTs) main purpose is to eliminate Mtb with minimal damage to the host [152]. HDTs include different groups of compounds, such as cytokines, repurposed-drugs that target biologically and clinically relevant checkpoints in anti-Mtb-directed host response pathways [152].

Macrophages are derived from monocyte precursors and undergo specific differentiation depending on the local tissue environment. M1 (IFNγ/LPS) macrophages are characterized by production of pro-inflammatory mediators such as nitric oxide (NO) usually associated with the control of infection [153]. In contrast, M2 (IL-4/IL-13) macrophages are immune modulators by secreting more ornithine and support a Th2-associated effector function [153]. Mtb has evolved different strategies to interfere with M1 (IFNγ/LPS) polarization, neutralize microbicidal effectors to promote M2 (IL-4/IL-13) polarization resulting in its persistence and survival in the macrophages [153]. Effective immune defence against invading pathogens is dependent on a wide transcriptional program in macrophages and other immune cells [18]. Factors such as chromatin remodelling, transcription factor activation, receptor ligation and signalling all coordinate the duration and intensity of these responses [18]. While the role of miRNAs in the regulation of inflammatory responses has been well studied [154], the role of long noncoding RNAs in polarized macrophages and during infection with infectious pathogens is still poorly understood.

In this study, we demonstrate that MIR99AHG is highly upregulated by IL-4/IL-13 stimulation and downregulated by Mtb infection in macrophages. Using loss-of-function approach, we gained insights into the biological functions of MIR99AHG at both cellular level and organismal level. Knockdown of MIR99AHG reduced intracellular Mtb growth in mouse and human macrophages and induced apoptosis. Knockdown of MIR99AHG reduced pro-inflammatory cytokines such as IL-6 and IL-1β. Knockdown of MIR99AHG impaired the expression of the neighbouring gene coxsackie virus and adenovirus receptor (Cxadr) suggesting a *cis*-regulatory role. Our mechanistic studies also show that MIR99AHG functions through is interaction with hnRNPA2/B1. The evidence from the fractional RNA extraction reveals that MIR99AHG is translocated to the nucleus post IL-4/IL-13 stimulation.

MIR99AHG was previously identified and referred to as MONC [29]. MIR99AHG was reported to be spliced into a 710-nucleotide lincRNA, where intron 6 of MONC produces the miRNAs MIR99A, LET7C and MIR125B2 [29]. Emmrich *et al.* [29] found that knockdown of MIR99AHG in AMKL cell lines with high endogenous MIR99AHG expression reduced cell growth and colony-forming capacity [29]. Knockdown of MIR99AHG induced apoptosis and changed megakaryocytic-erythroid surface markers in a cell-line dependent manner [29]. Our findings show similarity to what was reported [29], suggesting that MIR99AHG may function in a similar manner to other disease models. This is further supported by the observed downregulation of MIR99AHG by other intracellular pathogens (Figure S2C-E).

Knockdown of MIR99AHG reduced Mtb intracellular growth and induced apoptosis in both mouse and human macrophages (Figure 2C-D and Figure 8C). The way macrophages respond following Mtb infection is very crucial to the host immune response and the outcome of the infection. Apoptosis is one of the major outcomes observed following established Mtb infection in macrophages and an important host defence mechanism [155]. It has been reported that apoptosis is able to control bacterial growth, however virulent strains of Mtb have been reported to inhibit the completion of apoptosis [156]. This is a virulence mechanism used by the pathogen to escape host defences, and results in necrosis and persistent infection of the surrounding macrophages [156]. Our results suggest that apoptosis is used as a host defence mechanism to control Mtb infection. The secretion of pro-inflammatory cytokines is very important in the protection against Mtb infection. To maintain control of Mtb infection cytokines such as IFNγ, TNFα, IL-6, IL-1β are needed [157]. We sought to examine whether knocking down MIR99AHG would have any altered effect on the above-mentioned cytokine production given their role in the control of Mtb infection. Knockdown of MIR99AHG reduced the production of IL-6 and IL-1β in M2 (IL-4/IL-13) and Mtb infected macrophages suggesting that MIR99AHG may be a positive regulator of inflammation. Quite a few long noncoding RNAs have been reported to be important regulators of inflammation or act as "brakes" in controlling excessive inflammation [13, 14, 16, 158]. Our results suggest that MIR99AHG may play a crucial role as a potential regulator of macrophage polarization and inflammation while Mtb manipulates the host response by downregulating MIR99AHG to enable its survival in macrophages.

An important finding in our study is that MIR99AHG has a *cis* effect on its neighbouring gene Cxadr. Cxadr is an important cellular protein that is involved in cell-adhesion, protein trafficking and viral infection [159]. Most lncRNAs have been reported as *trans*-acting regulators of protein-coding genes, such as *lincRNA-COX2* [14] and *NEAT1* [160]. While the importance of *trans*-acting lncRNAs in regulating immune response is highlighted in these studies, there remains a gap in the role of *cis*-regulatory lncRNAs in immune responses. A recent study published by Zhang and colleagues [158] identified a *cis*-acting lncRNA named *ROCKI* which regulates inflammatory gene expression. Regulation of gene expression by *cis*-acting lncRNAs may involve regulatory components in gene promoters, the process of transcription or splicing, or the sequence /structure of the RNAs [161]. However, many studies have shown that *cis*-regulatory functions of lncRNAs were dependent on sequence/structure of RNAs [162, 163]. Our study identifies MIR99AHG as a *cis*-regulatory lncRNA and further adds support to the role of *cis*-acting lncRNAs in immune regulation.

There are increasing studies of lncRNAs that have been functionally characterized especially in cancer models, however there is limited data on characterized lncRNAs in a TB disease model. Mouse models that use genetic deletion or antibody inhibition have shown an association between components of the immune system and survival upon Mtb challenge

[164]. Studies that have been performed on mouse models have also corresponded with observation made in humans hence data from mouse models is very crucial on improving current therapeutic interventions [164]. TB animal models are crucial for developing biomarkers of diagnosis, drug therapy, vaccines and for researching mechanisms that identify targets [165]. Recent studies have shown strong evidence on the role of lncRNAs in the modulation of innate and adaptive immune response. Findings from animal models, using systemic administration of antisense oligonucleotides (ASO), serve as a translational proof of concept for therapeutic interventions targeting lncRNAs [166]. In this study, we provide evidence for the regulation of immunity to Mtb by MIR99AHG. We explored the role of MIR99AHG in a loss of function approach. We used Mtb-infected mice systemically administered with LNA GapmeRs in comparison to infected negative control (NC) mice. Interestingly, MIR99AHG KD mice were highly resistant to TB disease exhibiting reduced tissue inflammation and pulmonary histopathology. We also show there is increased Caspase-3, a marker for apoptosis, in MIR99AHG KD group compared to the control. These results are consistent with our *in vitro* data. Unfortunately, we could not detect Arg1 on both groups at 3 weeks post infection. A study which showed that IL-4Rα does not play a significant role in TB disease progression also showed that Arg1 was not yet produced in the lungs of mice at four weeks post Mtb infection suggesting that Arg1 is induced at a later stage of infection [144]. Many studies have shown that miRNAs are involved in host responses to Mtb [167, 168], however there is limited research on the functional role of lncRNAs involved in host responses to Mtb infection. We show for the first time that treatment with MIR99AHG ASOs significantly reduced the pathogenesis of Mtb infection, suggesting that MIRR9AHG could be repurposed for host-directed therapy for TB.

Our mechanistic studies indicate that MIR99AHG functions by interacting with hnRNPA2/B1. Interestingly, this protein has been identified to interact with *lincRNA-COX2* [14]. hnRNPs are important functional partners for many additional lncRNAs. These include *lincRNA-EPS* which interacts with hnRNPL [13], *lincRNA-p21* which interacts with hnRNPK [169] and *Xist* which interacts with hnRNPU [170]. hnRNPs are well known to be involved in mRNA biogenesis. In addition, the role of hnRNPA2/B1 in transcriptional regulation of gene expression is also beginning to emerge. For example, hnRNPA2/B1 was shown to interact with small activating dsRNA to induce transcriptional activation [171]. Moreover, hnRNPA2/B1 regulates smooth muscle cell (SMC) differentiation gene expression transcriptionally and promotes neural crest cell migration and differentiation toward SMC [172]. Although in this study we show that MIR99AHG interacts with hnRNPA2/B1, more studies to substantiate this claim are needed. The identification of hnRNPA2/B1 as a functional binding partner of MIR99AHG adds further support to the role of hnRNPs in transcriptional regulation and expanding the role of these binding proteins beyond their well-known functions in mRNA processing.

RT-qPCR on fractionated RNA showed a nuclear localization of MIR99AHG. In the nucleus, it is most likely that RNAs play an important role in the organization of nuclear domains [173]. LncRNAs control the epigenetic state of particular genes, participate in transcriptional regulation, involved in alternative splicing and constitute subnuclear compartments [173]. In the nucleus, lncRNAs can act in *cis* or *trans*, for example *Morrbid* interacts with PRC2 to repress transcription of the neighbouring gene, Bim (*Bcl2l11*), in *cis* in short-lived myeloid cells such a s neutrophils and monocytes [174]. A lncRNA can interact with its protein partner as a guide (lincRNA:hnRNPL) [13], scaffold (RMRP interaction with DDX5 and RORγt) [175] or decoy molecule (Lethe:NF-κB p65) [176] to mediate its molecular functions. Cellular localization of lncRNAs can help with studies involving functions and mechanisms of action. Further studies in identifying the exact sub-nuclear areas and DNA target sequences of MIR99AHG are needed.

3.4 Conclusion
In conclusion, this study functionally validates for the first time the role of MIR99AHG during Mtb infection. MIR99AHG plays a role in the regulation of inflammatory genes, neighbouring gene and Mtb persistence in macrophages. In active TB patients, and Mtb-infected mice and human macrophages. MIR99AHG contributes to the maintenance of Mtb growth. Identifying the role of MIR99AHG during Mtb infection will ultimately provide a novel treatment approach for host-directed drug therapy for TB.

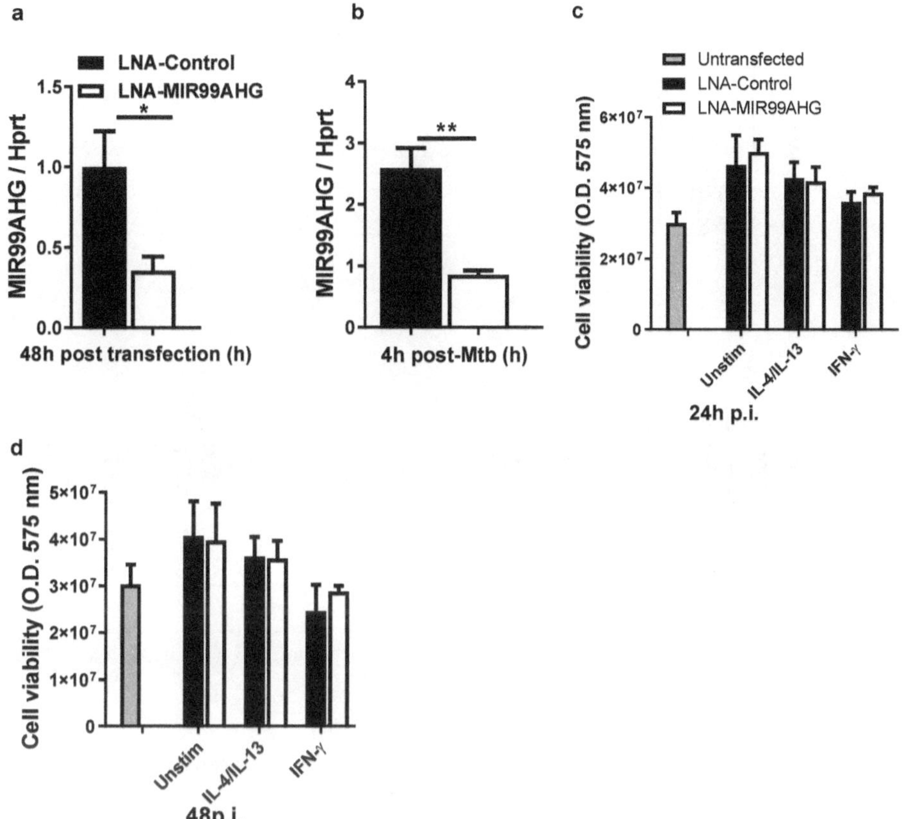

Figure S1. Knockdown efficiency and cell viability following LNA GapmeR treatment. (A, B) Knockdown efficiency of MIR99AHG on LNA GapmeR transfected BMDMs at 48 hours post transfection and 4 hours post Mtb infection, analysed by RT-qPCR. **(C, D)** Cell viability of LNA GapmeR transfected BMDMs at 24-72 hours post Mtb infection. Error bars denote mean ± SD. Data shown are representative of three independent experiments. *$P<0.05$, **$P<0.01$, ****$P<0.0001$, Student's *t*-test.

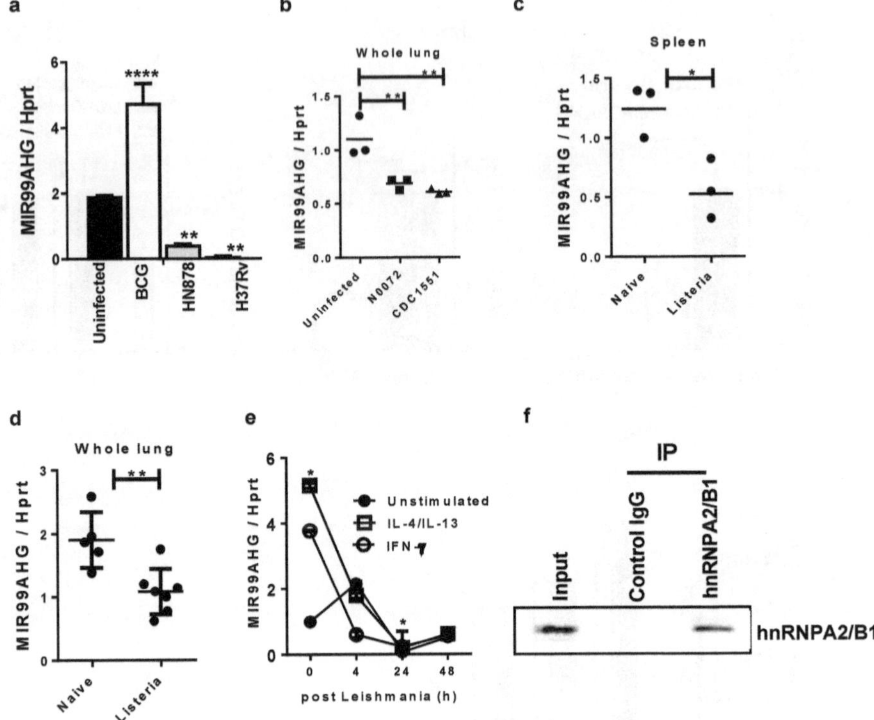

Figure S2. MIR99AHG is suppressed by other intracellular pathogens. (A) BMDMs were pre-stimulated with IL-4/IL-13 for 4 hours then infected with different Mtb strains for 24 hours to measure MIR99AHG mRNA by RT-qPCR. Error bars denote mean ± SD of triplicates. Two-way ANOVA and Bonferroni post-hoc test was used to analyse the statistical significance. Data shown are representative of one experiment.

(B) MIR99AHG mRNA expression measured by RT-qPCR in whole lung from wild-type mice infected with different Mtb strains (100 CFU/mouse) for 11 days. Error bars denote mean ± SD of triplicates. Two-way ANOVA and Bonferroni post-hoc test was used to analyse the statistical significance. Data shown are representative of one experiment.

(C, D) MIR99AHG mRNA expression measured by RT-qPCR in whole lung and spleen from wild-type mice infected with *Listeria monocytogenes* (2×10^5 CFU/mouse) at 2 dpi. Error bars denote mean ± SD of triplicates. Data shown are representative of one experiment.

(E) Expression of MIR99AHG mRNA measured by RT-qPCR from BMDMs pre-stimulated with IFN-γ or IL-4/IL-13 for 4 hours and infected with *Leishmania mexicana*. Error bars denote mean ± SD of triplicates. Data shown are representative of three independent experiments.

(F) Western blot analysis of hnRNPA2/B1 in Input and anti-hnRNPA2/B1 antibody immunoprecipitates from LNA-MIR99AHG knockdown macrophages stimulated with IL-4/IL-13 and infected with Mtb. Bands were cut from previous experiments. P values represented as, *$P<0.05$, **$P<0.01$ and ***$P<0.0001$, Student's *t*-test.

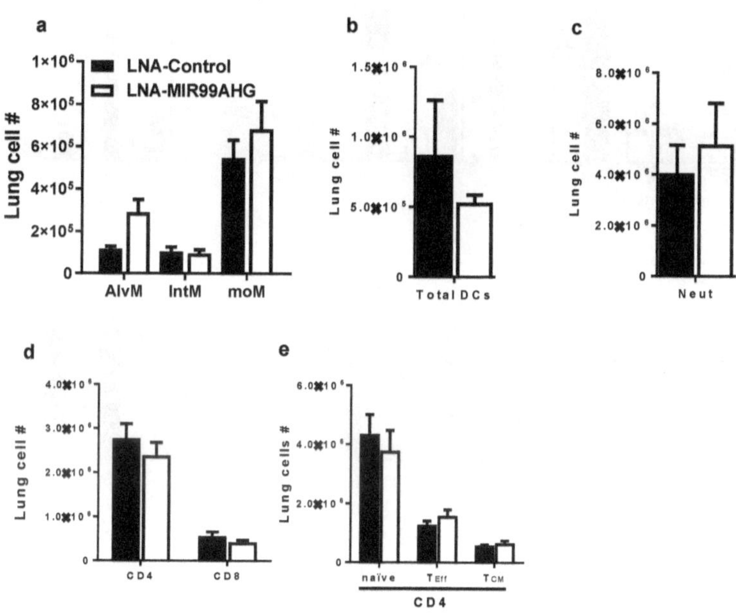

Figure S3. Lung myeloid and lymphoid cell numbers in cell populations following Mtb HN878 infection in MIR99AHG knockdown mice. Mice were LNA GapmeR treated with negative control and MIR99AHG at 10 mg/kg for alternative days up to day 14. Mice were infected intranasally with 100 CFU/mouse of Mtb HN878 (n=6 mice/group) and sacrificed at 3 weeks post-infection. **(A)** Cell numbers of lung CD11c+SiglecF+autofluorescence[high] alveolar macrophages (AlvM), lung CD11b+ F4/80+Ly6G- interstitial recruited macrophages (IntM) and CD11b+CD64+CD11c-monocyte-derived macrophages (moM); **(B)** lung CD11b+CD11c+MHCII+CD103- Ly6C- and lung CD11b-CD103+CD11c+ DC; **(C)** lung CD11b+Ly6G+

neutrophils. **(D, E)** Cell numbers of lung lymphoid CD3$^+$CD4$^+$, CD3$^+$CD8$^+$ T cells, CD44^{low}CD62L^{high} naïve CD4+, effector CD44^{high}CD62L^{low} CD4$^+$ T cells and central memory CD44^{high}CD62L^{high} CD4$^+$. Data representative of one experiment.

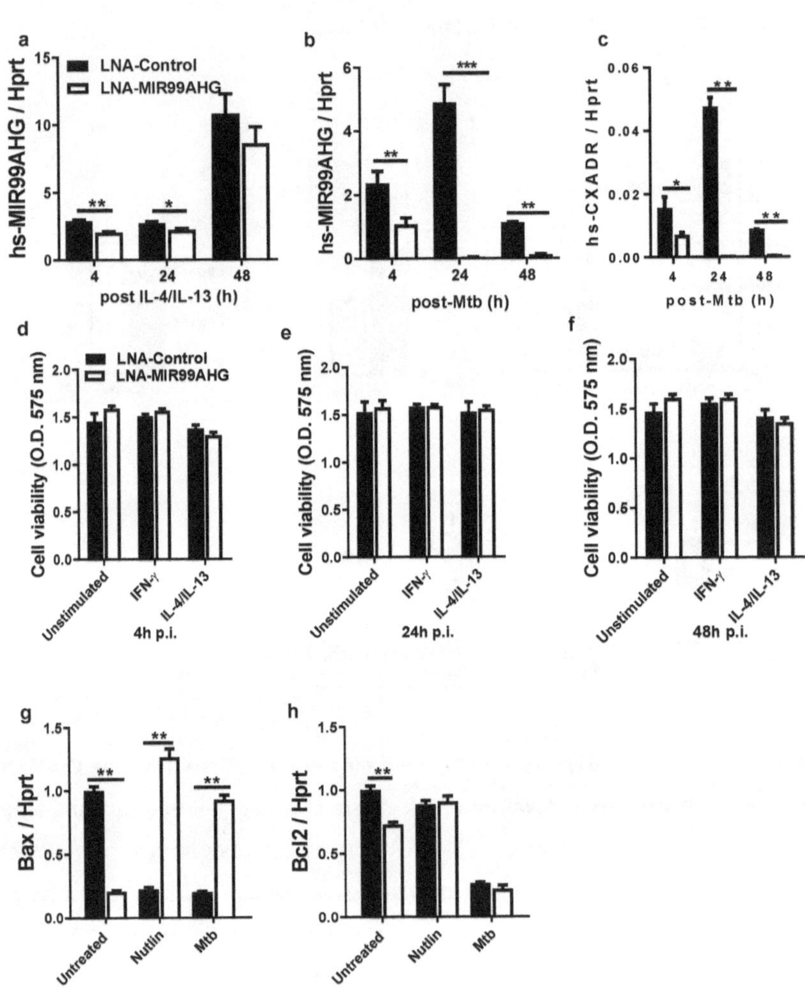

Figure S4. Knockdown efficiency MIR99AHG following LNA GapmeR treatment in human MDMs. (A-C) Human MIR99AHG and CXADR knockdown efficiency on human MDMs pre-stimulated by IL-4/IL-13 for 4 hours and infected with Mtb HN878, analysed by RT-qPCR. Error bars denote mean ± SD. Data shown are representative of three independent experiments. **(D-F).** Cell viability of LNA GapmeR transfected human MDMs pre-stimulated with IL-4/IL-13 for 4 hours and infected with Mtb for 4 to 48 hours. Error bars denote mean ± SD. Data shown are representative of one experiment.

(G, H). Bax and Bcl2 mRNA expression measured by RT-qPCR from LNA GapmeR transfected human MDMs treated with nutlin, rapamycin and Mtb infection for 24 hours. Error bars denote mean ± SD of triplicates. Data shown are representative of one experiment. P values represented as, *$P<0.05$, **$P<0.01$ and ****$P<0.0001$, Student's *t*-test.

Chapter 4: IL7-AS promotes Mtb intracellular growth through regulation of inflammatory genes

4.1 Introduction

Mycobacterium tuberculosis (Mtb) remains the leading bacterial cause of death in humans worldwide (1.5 million deaths per year) [1]. Mtb is predominantly transmitted by the respiratory route, and while it is able to cause disease in most organs in the body, the most reported and occurring is pulmonary tuberculosis where it establishes its niche within macrophages [8]. The innate system is the first defence against invading pathogens through activating inflammatory responses [177]. Macrophages, dendritic cells and neutrophils are known to play important roles as antigen presenting cells (APCs) in the innate host defence [8].

Long non-coding RNAs were initially identified in mice through FANTOM project [178]. Long non-coding RNAs (lncRNAs) are mainly classified as either short noncoding RNA (< 200 nucleotides) or long noncoding RNA (> 200 nucleotides) [10]. LncRNAs are classified according to their position to protein coding genes which include antisense (AS), long intergenic (lincRNA) and pseudogenes [10]. Many of these lncRNAs are commonly induced post activation of the innate immune response [179]. LncRNAs have emerged as key regulators of chromatin remodelling, transcription and posttranscriptional gene regulation in the innate immune system [180].

Recent publications have identified several lncRNAs that are differentially expressed following activation of the innate immune response which leads to subsequent regulation of inflammatory response. Many studies in mice have identified *lincRNA-Cox2* [14, 58], *lincRNA-EPS* [13], *Mirt2* [16] and *IL7-AS* [30], while in humans these include *THRIL* [15], *IL7-AS* [31], *lnc-IL7R* [43] and *IL1β-RBT* [181]. LncRNA IL7-AS is newly discovered and has been reported to be located antisense to IL-7 and induced in many mice and human cell types following exposure to LPS or IL-1β [31]. Knockdown of IL7-AS was shown to not have a significant effect on the mRNA expression of IL-7 in A549, THP-1 and RAW264.7 cell lines [31]. Another publication has shown that IL7-AS is differentially expressed in human lung fibroblasts following IL-1β induction to negatively regulate IL-6 [179]. Recently, this lncRNA has been shown to be dependent on the NF-κB and MAPK signalling pathways in macrophages and epithelial cells and also induce the expression of CCL2, CCL5 and CCL7 [182].

There are few publications that have shown the functional role of lncRNAs during Mtb infection [64, 68]. However, despite the role of these lncRNAs during Mtb infection and following the activation of the innate immune response, there has been no attempt to identify the role of lncRNAs in polarised macrophages and/or during Mtb infection. To address this issue, we determined the functional role of lncRNA IL7-AS in mouse and human polarized macrophages and during Mtb infection. In this study we show that IL7-AS is highly induced following Mtb infection. IL7-AS appears to negatively regulate IL-6, IL-1α, IL-1β and IL-12 in Mtb infected macrophages. Knockdown of IL7-AS does not seem to have a significant impact on the mRNA production of IL-7 suggesting that the function if IL7-AS is not dependent on IL-7 *in cis*. We also show that it is dependent on the NF-κB and MAPK signalling pathways in macrophages. We show the relevance of IL7-AS in active TB patients and in human macrophages. Therefore, our data show an important role of IL7-AS as a promoter of Mtb growth and transcriptional activator of inflammatory genes during Mtb infection.

4.2 Results
4.2.1 IL7-AS is induced following Mtb infection
Using the same approach to identify *lincRNA-MIR99AHG*, we utilized CAGE transcriptomics to identify IL-7AS from activated BMDMs [142] and during Mtb infection [147]. From this approach we identified several differentially expressed lncRNAs that were either upregulated or downregulated in polarized and/or Mtb infected BMDMs. We chose IL7-AS because it was highly upregulated by Mtb, an opposite effect to what we observed with *lincRNA-MIR99AHG*. BMDMs were either stimulated towards an M1 (IFN-γ) or M2 (IL-4, IL-13, IL-4/IL-13) phenotype and/or infected with Mtb HN878 hypervirulent strain (Figure 4.1A). IL7-AS was one of the two lncRNAs that is upregulated by Mtb infection from our top 9 validated list of lncRNAs. There was no clear indication of which macrophage polarization phenotype had the most effect on IL7-AS, however upon Mtb infection we could observe a drastic upregulation of IL7-AS. (Figure 4.1B-C). Mtb infection upregulated 150 fold the TPM expression of IL7-AS compared to the unstimulated macrophages (Figure 4.1C). The expression of IL7-AS post stimulation and Mtb infection was confirmed by RT-qPCR (Figure 4.1D-E).

4.2.2 Knockdown of IL7-AS reduces intracellular Mtb growth through apoptosis and regulation of the transcription of inflammatory genes

To understand and validate the role of IL7-AS during Mtb infection we performed functional experiments on BMDMs and human MDMs using Locked Nucleic Acid (LNA) chemically engineered antisense oligonucleotides (ASOs) known as LNA GapmeRs. To examine the functional role of IL7-AS on intracellular growth of Mtb in macrophages, we inhibited IL7-AS using LNA antisense oligonucleotides (ASOs). The knockdown efficiency was at 60% and 53% at 24 and 48 hours post transfection, respectively (Figure 4.2A).

Cell viability was confirmed using Cell-Titre blue assay (Figure 4.2C). Next, we examined the functional role IL7-AS during Mtb infection by analysing its effect on the intracellular survival of Mtb by CFU assays. Knockdown of IL7-AS drastically reduced intracellular bacterial growth in unstimulated BMDMs (Figure 4.2B). By RT-qPCR we confirmed that knockdown of IL7-AS increased apoptosis in BMDMs treated with nutlin, an apoptosis inducer, and post Mtb infection by measuring mRNA levels of Bax and Bcl-2 (Figure 4.2D). To further characterize IL7-AS, we performed ELISA from BMDMs infected with Mtb. Knockdown of IL7-AS increased protein levels of IL-1α, IL-1β, IL-6 and IL-12 compared to the control (Figure 4.2E-I). We performed a Griess reagent assay and arginase assay to measure nitrite and arginase production post Mtb infection. Knockdown of IL7-AS increased nitrite production while there was no effect on arginase production (Figure 4.2J-K). These results suggest apoptosis enhancement and heightened pro-inflammatory gene response might account for the mechanisms behind the reduced intracellular Mtb growth. These data also suggest that Mtb targets IL7-AS to favour Mtb growth and persistence within the host.

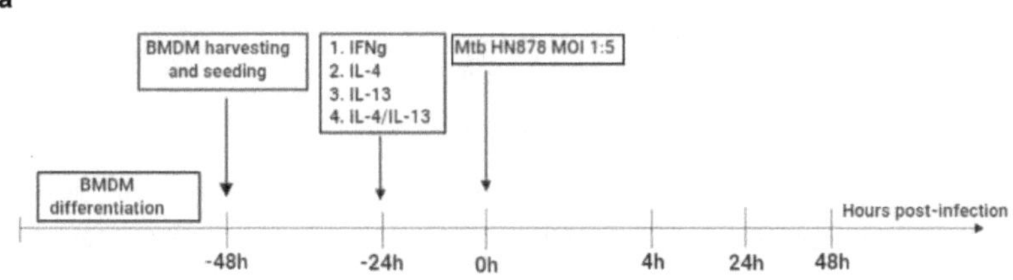

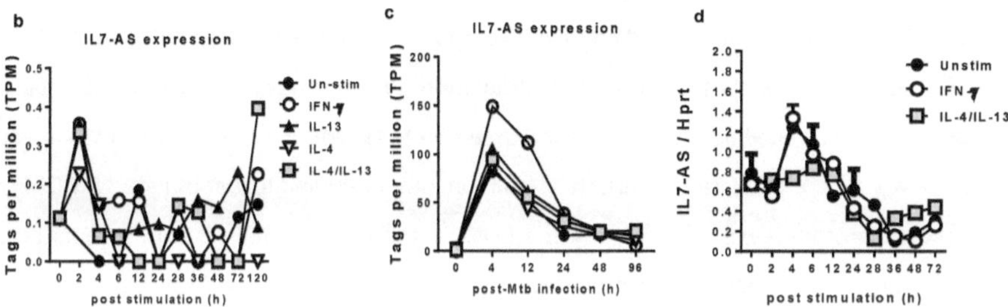

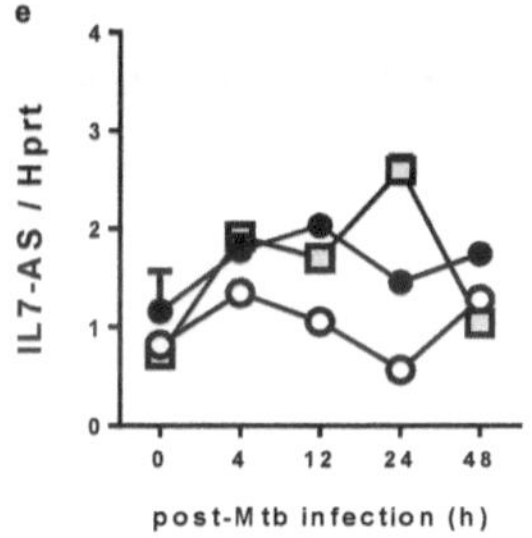

Figure 4.1 IL7-AS is highly induced by Mtb infection. (A) Timeline of mouse macrophage activation and Mtb HN878 infection. Bone marrow cells were differentiated for 10 days into BMDMs and stimulated with IFNγ or IL-4, IL-13, IL-4/IL-13. At 24 hours post-stimulation, BMDMs were infected with Mtb (HN878) for 4, 24 and 48 hours. RNA was extracted from lysed cells at different time points post-stimulation and post-Mtb infection. **(B, C)** CAGE analysis of IL7-AS kinetic expression in non-infected and Mtb-infected BMDMs. The fold change in gene expression was determined by RT-qPCR and was normalised to HPRT expression. Three independent experiments were performed.

(D, E) RT-qPCR analysis of IL7-AS kinetic expression in stimulated and Mtb-infected BMDMs. Data is representative of three independent experiments. Each data point represents arithmetic mean of triplicates ± SD of triplicates.

4.2.3 IL7-AS functions independently of IL-7

The mouse and human homologs of IL7-AS were renamed as a result of their antisense overlap with the promoter region of IL-7, a cytokine which is known to play an important role in B and T cell development [183]. To confirm whether knockdown of IL7-AS has any regulatory effects on the expression of IL-7, we performed RT-qPCR on BMDMs. Knockdown of IL7-AS increased the expression of IL-7 in a time dependent manner in unstimulated and Mtb infected BMDMs (Figure 4.3A-C). To determine whether loss of function of IL7-AS on BMDMS stimulated with IL-7 had any significant role in mycobacterial growth, we performed a CFU assay. Our results show that IL-7 stimulation does not have any significant impact on reducing Mtb intracellular growth in early time points except at 72 hours post Mtb infection (Figure 4.3D). We collected supernatant from unstimulated and IL-7 stimulated BMDMs and measured protein levels of IL-7 using the ELISA. Knockdown of IL7-AS in unstimulated and stimulated BMDMs increased protein levels of IL-7 in a negative regulatory manner (Figure 4.3E-F). Silencing of IL7-AS on BMDMs stimulated with IL-7 and Mtb infected did not have an impact on nitrite production however, arginase production was reduced (Figure 4.3G-H). These data suggest that despite the negative regulation of IL7-AS on IL-7, the intracellular Mtb growth is not due to the inhibition of IL-7 but rather on host factors such as pro-inflammatory cytokines.

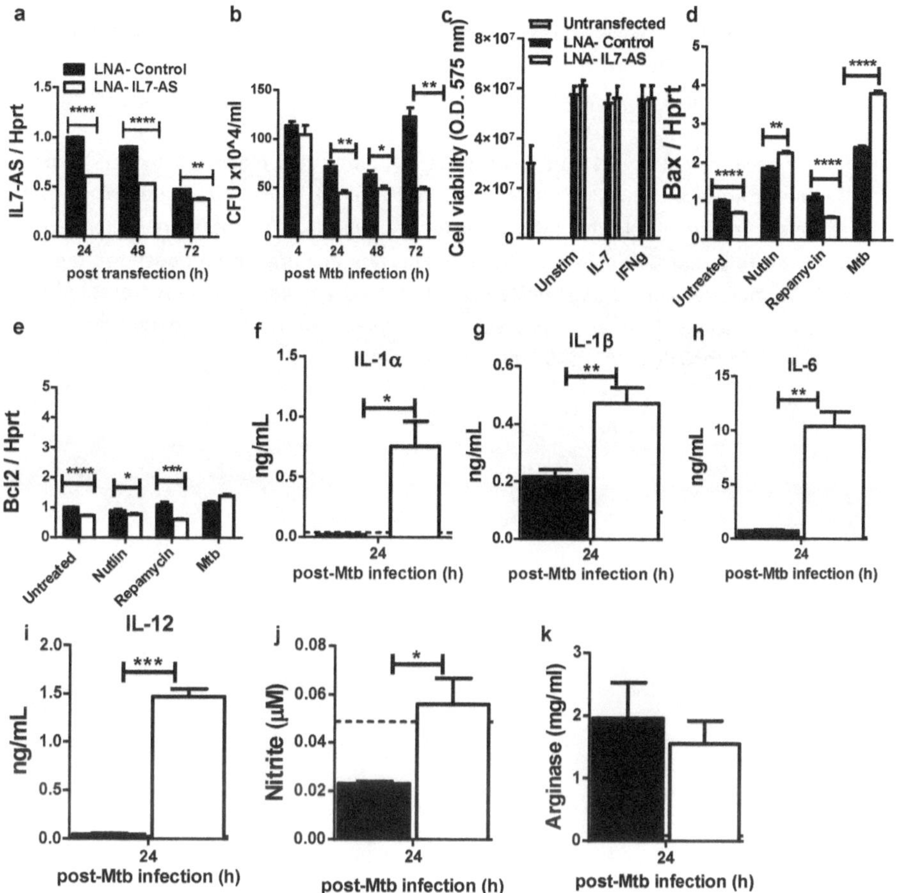

Figure 4.2 IL7-AS promotes Mtb growth by regulating the transcription of inflammatory genes.

(A) Knockdown efficiency of LNA-IL7-AS post LNA GapmeR transfection on BMDMs. Each data point represents arithmetic mean of triplicates ± SD. Three independent experiments were performed.

(B) BMDMs were LNA GapmeR transfected with LNA control and LNA IL7-AS and infected with Mtb. Cells were lysed at 4 hours for uptake and at 24 to 72 hours post-Mtb infection to measure bacterial growth by CFU counting. Each data point represents arithmetic mean of triplicates ± SD. Three independent experiments were performed.

(C) Cell viability of LNA-GapmeR transfected BMDMs at 4 hours post Mtb infection. Each data point represents arithmetic mean of triplicates ± SD. Three independent experiments were performed.

(D, E) Bax and Bcl2 mRNA expression measured by RT-qPCR from LNA-GapmeR transfected BMDMs treated with nutlin, rapamycin and Mtb infection for 24 hours. Each data point represents arithmetic mean of triplicates ± SD. Three independent experiments were performed.

(F, I) Protein cytokine levels of IL-1β, IL-1a, IL-12 and IL-6 measured by ELISA from LNA-GapmeR transfected BMDMs infected with Mtb for 24 hours. Each data point represents arithmetic mean of triplicates ± SD. Three independent experiments were performed.

(J, K) Nitrite production measured by Griess reagent and arginase production from BMDMs LNA-GapmeR transfected and infected with Mtb for 24 hours. Data are represented as mean ± SD of triplicates. Data are representative of three independent experiments.   *p<0.05, **p<0.01, ***p<0.001, ****p<0.0001, Student *t*-test.

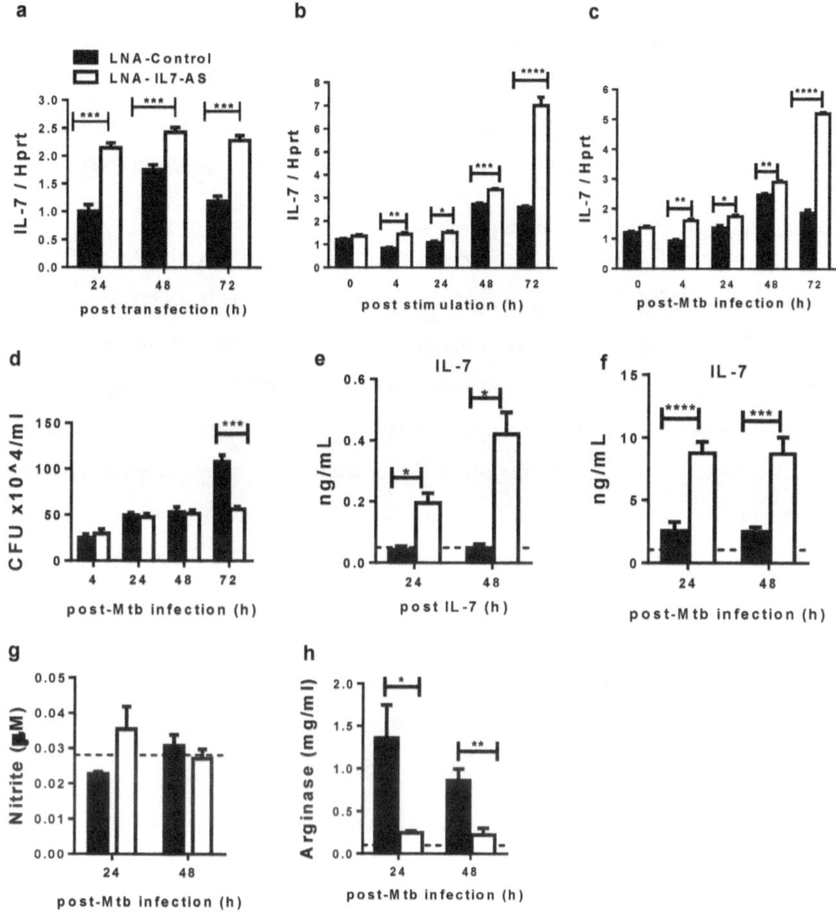

Figure 4.3 IL7-AS functions independently of IL-7. (A-C) IL-7 mRNA expression measured by RT-qPCR on BMDMs transfected with LNA-IL7-AS and LNA-Control, non-stimulated and infected with Mtb. Each data point represents arithmetic mean of triplicates ± SD. Three independent experiments were performed. **(D)** BMDMs were transfected with LNA control and LNA IL7-AS, stimulated with IL-7 and infected with Mtb. Cells were lysed at 4 hours for uptake and at 24-72 hours post-Mtb infection to measure bacterial growth by CFU counting. Each data point represents arithmetic mean of triplicates ± SD. Three independent experiments were performed. **(E, F)** Protein cytokine levels of IL-7 measured by ELISA from LNA-GapmeR transfected BMDMs stimulated with IL-7 and infected with Mtb. Each data point

represents arithmetic mean of triplicates ± SD. Three independent experiments were performed. **(G, H)** Nitrite production measured by Griess reagent and arginase production from BMDMs LNA-GapmeR transfected pre-stimulated with IL-7 and infected with Mtb. Data are represented as mean ± SD of triplicates. Data are representative of three independent experiments. *$P<0.05$, **$P<0.01$, ***$P<0.001$ and ****$P<0.0001$, Student's *t*-test.

4.2.4 IL7-AS is induced in Mtb infected mice

To examine the expression of IL7-AS *in vivo*, we collected whole lung from Mtb infected mice or naïve mice. IL7-AS was upregulated in mice infected with Mtb HN878 at 11 days post infection (Figure 4.4A). We observed the upregulation of IL7-AS from whole lung infected with Mtb clinical isolate CDC1551 and with the virulent N0072 strain (Figure 4.4B). We examined the expression of IL-7 which was upregulated at day 11 and 21 post infection (Figure 4.4C). We sorted by flow cytometry myeloid cells from Mtb infected lungs and naïve lungs and observed an upregulation of IL7-AS in interstitial recruiting macrophages, CD11DCs and neutrophils compared to the naïve cells (Figure 4.4D). As IL7-AS exhibits upregulated expression upon LPS stimulation *in vitro*, we challenged BALB/c mice with LPS at a sub-lethal dose (5 mg/kg mice weight; i.p.) for 4 and 8 hours and IL7-AS mRNA levels from various tissues were measured by RT-qPCR. LPS challenged mice had significantly elevated levels of IL7-AS in the peritoneal fluid, spleen and liver (Figure 4.4E-G). These results suggest that Mtb and LPS play a pivotal role in regulating IL7-AS both *in vitro* and *in vivo*.

4.2.5 IL7-AS is induced in BMDMs exposed to TLR ligands and dependent on the Myd88 signalling pathway

We employed RT-qPCR to examine the kinetics of IL7-AS expression in BMDMs exposed to TLR ligands including LPS (TLR 4) and Pam3CSK4 (TLR2/1). The expression of IL7-AS was upregulated in both TLR ligands in a time dependent manner (Figure 4.5A-B). To evaluate the role of NF-κB and MAPK pathways we used selective pharmacological inhibitors for NF-κB (Bay11-7084), Erk1/2 (FR180204, extracellular signal-regulated kinase), Jnk (SP600125, c-Jun N-terminal kinase) and p38 (SB203580) to assess the functional consequences of inhibition of these pathways on IL7-AS expression. BMDMs stimulated with LPS in the presence of NF-κB and MAPK inhibitors showed a significant decrease in IL7-AS expression (Figure 4.5C-E). Similarly, BMDMs infected with Mtb in the absence of NF-κB and MAPK pathways had a significant reduction in IL7-AS expression (Figure4.5F-I). Next, we sought to measure the expression of IL7-AS in MYD88$^{-/-}$ BMDMs, since TLR4 signalling is dependent on MYD88 and

TRIFF [150]. IL7-AS expression was inhibited in MYD88$^{-/-}$ BMDMs at 4 and 24 hours post LPS stimulation (Figure 4.5J). Collectively, these results suggest that IL7-AS expression is regulated by the NF-κB and MAPK pathways.

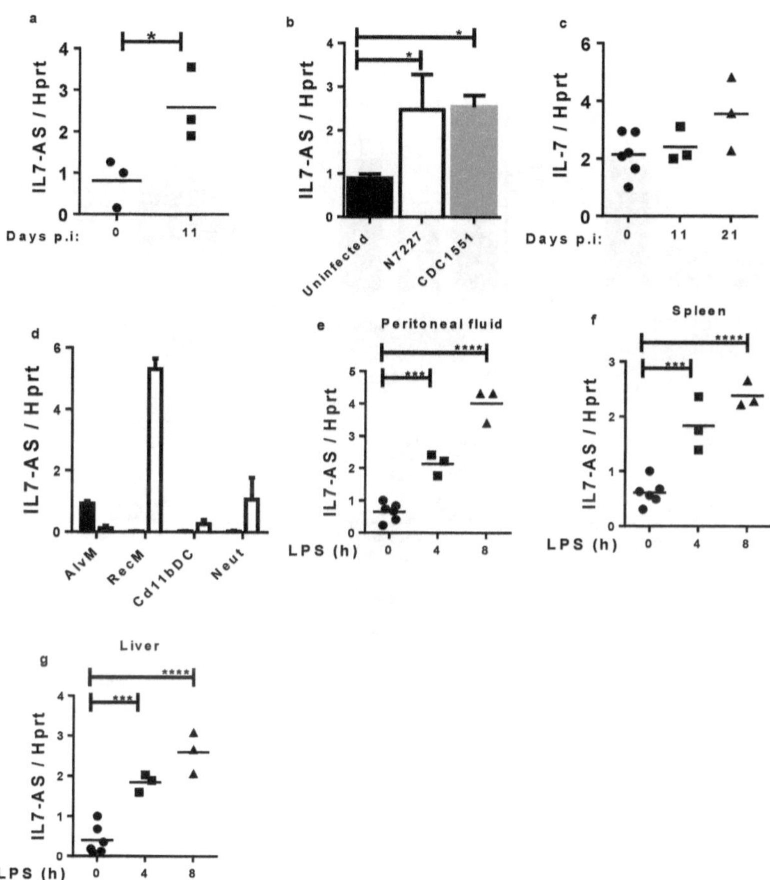

Figure 4.4 IL7-AS is induced by Mtb infection and LPS challenge *in vivo*. (A) IL7-AS mRNA expression measured by RT-qPCR on whole lung from wild-type (WT) mice infected with Mtb HN878 (100 CFU/mouse) for 11 days. **(B)** IL7-AS mRNA expression measured by RT-qPCR on whole lung from wild-type mice infected with different Mtb strains (100 CFU/mouse). **(C)** IL-7 mRNA expression measured by RT-qPCR on whole lung from wild type (WT) mice infected with Mtb HN878 (100 CFU/mouse) for 11 and 21 days. **(D)** IL7-AS mRNA expression measured by

RT-qPCR from myeloid sorted cells. **(E)** IL7-AS mRNA expression measured by RT-qPCR in peritoneal fluid, **(F)** spleen and **(G)** liver of WT mice challenged with LPS i.p. (5 mg/kg/mice) for 4 and 8 hours; n=3 mice per group. Data are represented as arithmetic mean of triplicates ± SD. Data are presentative of one experiment. P values represented as, *P<0.05, **P<0.01, ****P<0.0001, Student's t-test.

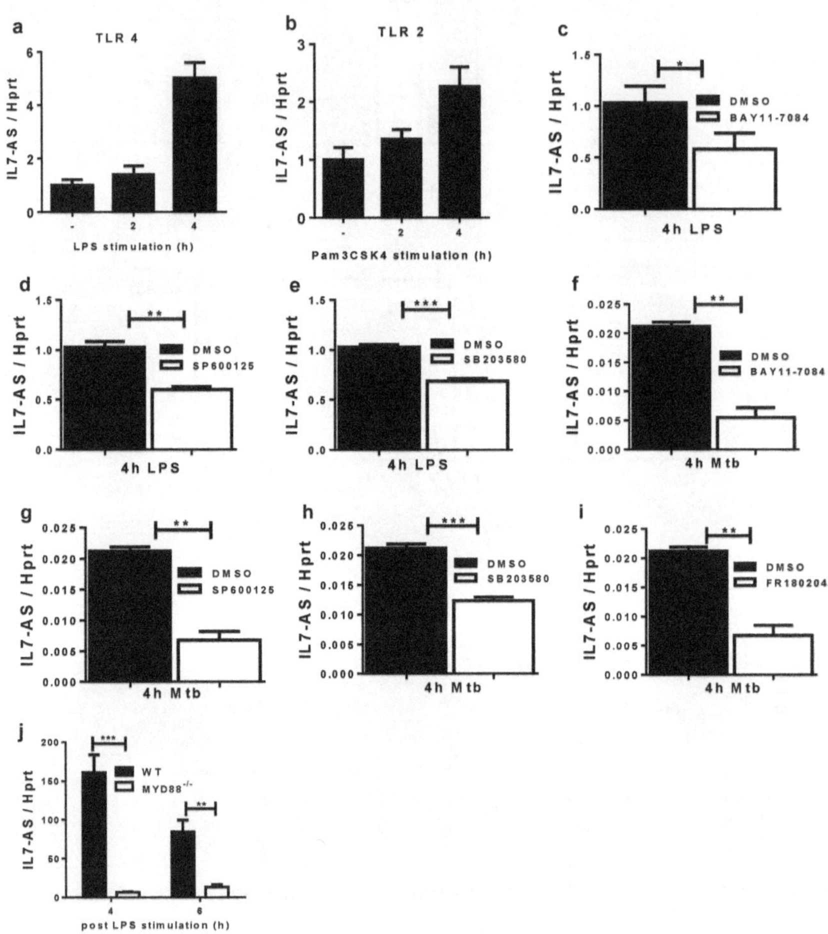

Figure 4.5 IL7-AS is induced in BMDMs exposed to TLR ligands and signals through Myd88. **(A, B)** RT-qPCR of IL7-AS mRNA expression in BMDMs stimulated with TLR-4 agonist LPS (100

ng/ml) and TLR-2 agonist Pam3Csk4 (100 ng/ml). Each data point represents arithmetic mean of triplicates ± SD. Three independent experiments were performed.

(C-E) BMDMs were pre-treated for 1 hour with selective pharmacological inhibitors for NF-κB (Bay11-7084, 10 µM), p38 (SB203580, 5 µM), Jnk (SP600125, 10 µM) and Erk1/2 (FR180204, 10 µM), then activated by LPS stimulation (100 ng/ml) for 4 hours. Each data point represents arithmetic mean of triplicates ± SD. Three independent experiments were performed, or

(F-I) Infected with Mtb HN878 for 4 hours. Expression of IL7-AS was detected by RT-qPCR. Data represents arithmetic mean of triplicates ± SD. Three independent experiments were performed.

(J) IL7-AS mRNA expression measured by RT-qPCR from MYD88$^{-/-}$ BMDMs stimulated with LPS. Data represents arithmetic mean of triplicates ± SD. Three independent experiments were performed. *$P<0.05$, **$P<0.01$ and ***$P<0.001$, Student's *t*-test.

4.2.6 IL7-AS is induced in Mtb-infected human macrophages and active TB patients

Because IL7-AS is conserved in humans as well, we observed its expression on human macrophages. We employed loss of function experiments using LNA GapmeRS to knockdown IL7-AS in human monocyte derived macrophages (MDMs). We confirmed knockdown efficiency of IL7-AS in unstimulated and LPS stimulated MDMs by RT-qPCR (Figure 4.6A-B). Knockdown of IL7-AS in human MDMs reduced Mtb intracellular growth at 24 and 48 hours post Mtb infection (Figure 4.6C). Knockdown of IL7-AS increased IL-6 protein levels measured by ELISA in unstimulated MDMs (Figure 4.6D). We examined IL7-AS and IL-7 expression from MDMs infected with Mtb HN878 *ex vivo*. Both IL7-AS and IL-7 were upregulated by Mtb infection in a time dependent manner (Figure4.6E-J). Finally, we collected PBMCs from healthy and active TB patients and re-stimulated with heat kill Mtb HN878. IL7-AS was upregulated in both active TB patients and re-stimulated PBMCs compared to healthy patients (Figure 4.6J-K). Taken together, these results show that IL7-AS is upregulated in human macrophages and in TB patients suggesting a possible target for host-directed therapy.

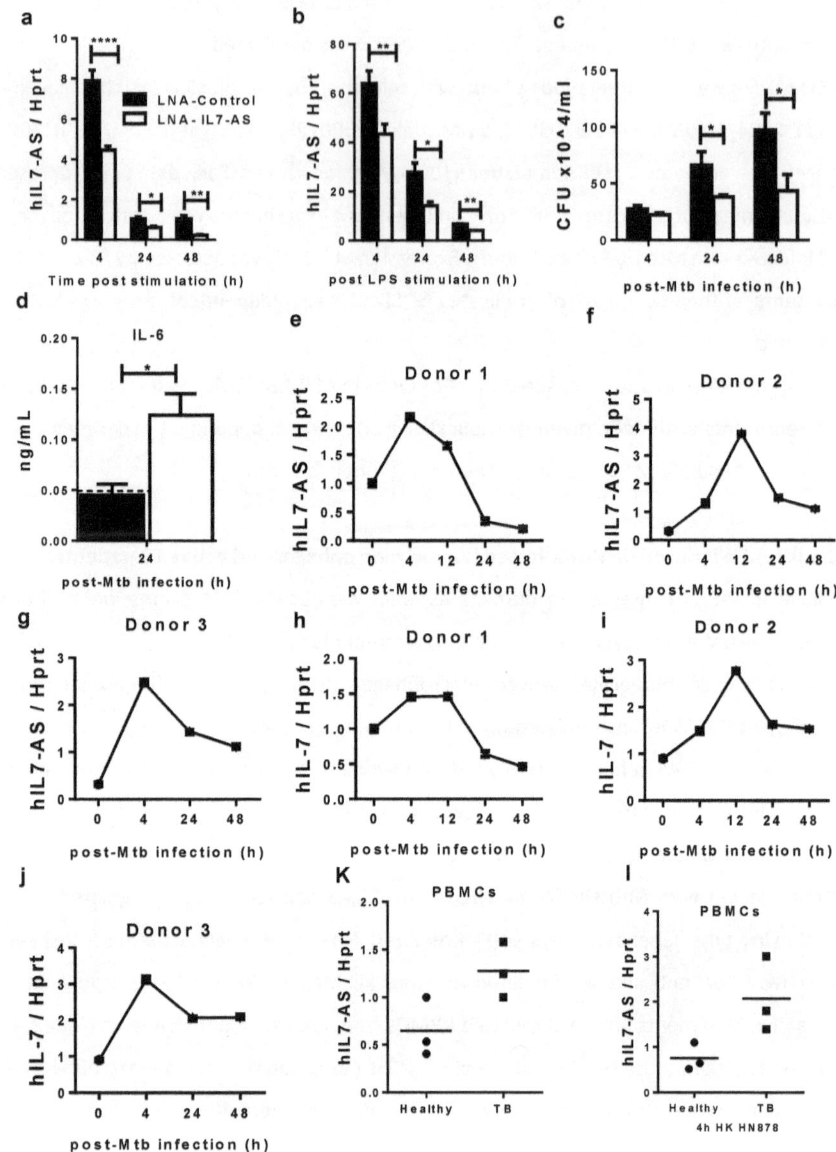

Figure 4.6 IL7-AS is induced in Mtb-infected human macrophages and active TB patients. (A, B) Knockdown efficiency of IL7-AS by LNA IL7-AS in unstimulated and LPS stimulated human

MDMs analysed by RT-qPCR. Data point represents arithmetic mean of triplicates ± SD. Three independent experiments were performed.

(C) MDMs were LNA GapmeR transfected for 48 hours and infected with Mtb HN878. Cells were lysed at 4h for uptake and at 24 and 48h post-Mtb infection to measure bacterial growth by CFU counting. Data represents arithmetic mean of triplicates ± SD. Three independent experiments were performed.

(D) IL-6 protein production measured by ELISA on LNA-GapmeR transfected MDMs infected with Mtb HN878 for 24 hours. Data represents arithmetic mean of triplicates ± SD. Three independent experiments were performed.

(E-G) RT-qPCR of IL7-AS mRNA expression on MDMs from healthy donors infected with Mtb HN878. Data represents arithmetic mean of triplicates ± SD. Three independent experiments were performed.

(H, J) RT-qPCR of IL-7 mRNA expression on MDMs from healthy donors infected with Mtb (HN878). Data point represents arithmetic mean of triplicates ± SD. Three independent experiments were performed.

(K, L) RT-qPCR of IL7-AS mRNA expression on re-stimulated PBMCs from healthy and active TB patients analysed by RT-qPCR. Data point represents arithmetic mean of triplicates ± SD. Data is representative of one experiment. P values represented as, *P<0.05, **P<0.01 and ***P<0.001, Student's *t*-test.

4.3 Discussion

Whilst the role of lncRNAs during Mtb infection remain unclear, there is growing research that indicates the association of lncRNAs with inflammation and regulation in the innate and adaptive immune response [12]. Using CAGE sequencing, we show for the first time differential lncRNA expression changes in polarised and Mtb infected mouse and human macrophages. This is very crucial since differential expression has always been the first step in identifying functional lncRNAs and has led to the identification of a number of lncRNAs that regulate inflammatory responses in immune cells including *lincRNA-EPS* [13], *lincRNA-Cox2* [14, 58], *lncRNA-Mirt2* [16] in mice and *THRIL* [15], *lnc-IL7R* [43] and *PACER* [184] in humans to mention a few. The CAGE approach enabled us to identify a recently annotated lncRNA, IL7-AS, that is induced across multiple human and murine cell types. IL-7-AS is transcribed antisense to IL-7 gene. IL7-AS was first identified in human monocytes stimulated with LPS using RNA sequencing [44]. Recently published studies have shown that IL7-AS is induced by LPS in human, mouse cell lines [31, 182] and IL-1β stimulated pulmonary lung fibroblasts [179]. These studies suggest that IL7-AS may have a significant role in the innate immune system.

In this study we observed no clear expression of IL7-AS in M0, M (IFN-γ) and M (IL-4/IL-13). Even though stimulation without Mtb showed no differential expression of IL7-AS, we did however observe a distinct upregulation of IL7-AS in Mtb infected macrophages. Because we did not see a distinct expression in M (IFN-γ) and M (IL-4/IL-13), we focused on M0 and Mtb infected macrophages for further functional validation. M1 (IFN-γ) macrophages are characterized by production of pro-inflammatory mediators such as nitric oxide (NO) usually associated with the control of infection [153]. In contrast, M2 (IL-4/IL-13) macrophages are immune modulators by secreting more ornithine and support a Th2-associated effector function [153]. Mtb is known to have evolved different strategies to interfere with M1 (IFN-γ) polarization, neutralize microbicidal effectors to promote M2 (IL-4/IL-13) polarization resulting in its persistence and survival in the macrophages [153]. In this study, we demonstrate that knockdown of IL7-AS reduces intracellular Mtb growth in both mouse and human macrophages, suggesting that this lncRNA may be a target for Mtb growth. We sought to understand the mechanism behind the reduced Mtb growth by looking at inflammatory responses and apoptosis. Our data shows that knockdown of IL7-AS upregulated protein levels of IL-6, IL-1β, IL-1α and IL-12. This is similar to what was reported in murine, human, cancer cell lines [31, 182] and in lung fibroblasts [179]. These results suggest that IL7-AS is a negative regulator of inflammatory response. IL-1β and IL-1α have been linked to the control of Mtb infection [185]. However it has been reported that IL-6 produced by Mtb-infected macrophages can contribute to the inability of the host cell response to eradicate the infection [186] and Mtb is able to manipulate host IL-6 production so as to decrease type 1 interferon signalling which leads to disease progression [187].

M (IFN-γ) macrophages produce cytotoxic nitric oxide which is detrimental to Mtb growth [8]. Notably we observed increased nitrite production in the knockdown macrophages which contributed to the reduced intracellular growth. It has been reported that apoptosis is able to control bacterial growth, however virulent strains of Mtb have been reported to inhibit the completion of apoptosis [156]. This is a virulence mechanism used by the pathogen to escape host defences, and results in necrosis and persistent infection of the surrounding macrophages [156]. Our results suggest that apoptosis and increased inflammatory responses are used as a host defence mechanism to control Mtb infection. These data suggest that Mtb targets IL7-AS to increase Mtb intracellular growth by regulating inflammatory genes and apoptosis.

IL-7 is known to be important for T and B cell development [188]. IL-7 which signals through the IL-7R plays a critical role in promoting T-cell survival by upregulating the expression of anti-apoptotic genes Bcl-2 and Mcl-1 [189]. Knockdown of IL7-AS did have a significant impact on IL-7 mRNA and protein levels indicating that IL7-AS controls the expression of IL-7 either directly in *cis* or indirectly in *trans*, given that IL7-AS knockdown also affects the expression of other inflammatory cytokines. IL-7 treatment in mice infected with LCMV is reported to increase cytokine production of IL-6, IL-1β, IL-1α, TNFα and CCL5 [190]. IL-7 was also shown to upregulate IL-8 mRNA expression in resting and human blood monocytes stimulated with LPS, IL-1β and TNF-α [191]. Here, we show that the Mtb growth-promoting effect of IL7-AS is independent of its inhibition of IL-7 expression since stimulating BMDMs with IL-7 following IL7-AS knock down (50% efficiency) does not yield a synergistic further reduction of Mtb growth in BMDMs. The treatment of murine macrophages with IL-7 infected with *Leishmania major* significantly cleared leishmanial infection [192]. The survival of Mtb infected mice has been shown to be enhanced by IL-7 treatment in BALB/c mice 3 weeks post infection [193]. This is like our results where we observed reduced intracellular Mtb growth in BMDMs treated with IL-7 then infected with Mtb.

TLR 2 and TLR 4 are known to play pivotal roles in the induction of immune response to many different infectious disease including *Mycobacterium* species [194]. TLR 2 is known to mediate Mtb-induced TNF-α expression, while TLR 4 plays significant role in the resistance to Mtb infection [194]. The activation of MAPK pathways leads to the induction of transcription factors including NF-Kb [195]. All three MAPK pathways are activated post Mtb infection and linked to disease pathogenesis [196]. Promoter binding of transcription factors may regulate lncRNA gene expression. In this study, we show that IL7-AS is induced by both TLR 2 and TLR 4 and dependent on the NF-κB and MAPK signalling pathways. Many lncRNAs have been shown to be dependent on the NF-κB and MAPK pathways including p38, JNK and Erk1/2 [13]. Previous studies have shown that the promoter binding of the NF-kB p65 subunit and MAPK c-Jun subunit are both needed for the trans-activation of IL7-AS in macrophages and in epithelial cells post-LPS stimulation [182].

IL7-AS has been reported to be conserved in both mouse and human and induced in various cell types [31]. Our study revealed that knockdown of IL7-AS prompted reduction of Mtb intracellular growth and increased expression of IL-6 in human macrophages. This is similar to what was observed in our mouse data. These results imply that IL7-AS may be an important regulator in innate immune response. Additionally, we observed an upregulation of IL7-AS and IL-7 in human MDMs infected with Mtb and in PBMCs from active TB patients or re-stimulated with heat killed Mtb. Therefore, IL7-AS is a key factor not only in inflammatory responses but also in controlling Mtb infection progression.

In conclusion we functionally characterized IL7-AS, which is conserved in both mouse and human. IL7-AS is shown to be a target for Mtb growth and persistence by regulating inflammatory responses. IL7-AS is induced by Mtb and LPS and depends on the NF-κB and MAPK pathways. An experiment where we assess the role of IL7-AS in the pathogenesis of TB *in vivo* is crucial. The role of IL7-AS in TB pathogenesis and inflammatory gene response is very relevant to the development of new host directed therapeutic strategies aimed at treating TB disease.

Chapter 5: General discussion and conclusions

5.1 Aim for chapter 3
The aim of this book was to functionally validate lincRNA-MIR99AHG and its interacting partner in polarized and/or Mtb-infected macrophages using chemically engineered antisense oligonucleotides (GapmeRs). To carry out this investigation, we performed knockdown experiments of MIR99AHG in mice and human macrophages as well *in vivo* using antisense oligonucleotides.

5.2 Summary of results from Chapter 3
Our work on the functional role of MIR99AHG was presented in Chapter 3. Following stimulation and Mtb infection in M1 (IFNγ) and M2 (IL-4/IL-13) macrophages, we observed an upregulation of MIR99AHG in M2 (IL-4/IL-13) macrophages and a downregulation upon Mtb infection. These results suggest that MIR99AHG is induced in M2 (IL-4/IL-13) macropahges and inhibited by Mtb. Knockdown of MIR99AHG in both mouse and human macrophages resulted in reduced intracellular Mtb growth and proinflammatory genes such as IL-6 and IL-1β. The production of nitrite and CD86 was reduced compared to the control. Knockdown of MIR99AHG led to increased apoptosis measured by flow cytometry suggesting that apoptosis and not proinflammatory gene induction is the mechanism underlying the reduced Mtb growth. MIR99AHG was also confirmed to have a *cis*-regulatory effect on the nearby gene, Cxadr. To investigate whether the beneficial effects of MIR99AHG suppression could be translated into a host-directed therapy (HDT), we used antisense oligonucleotides known as LNA GapmeRs to knockdown (KD) MIR99AHG in a mouse Mtb infection model and tested its prophylactic efficacy. At 3 weeks post infection there was reduced mycobacterial load in the lungs and spleen of MIR99AHG KD mice compared to the control group. Lung inflammation measured by alveolar spaces was significantly increased in MIR99AHG KD mice. We also observed reduced neutrophil influx, iNOS and T cell recruitment in MIR99AHG KD mice compared to the control group. We did however notice increased apoptosis in Mtb infected mice treated with MIR99AHG *in vivo* as also measured in human and mouse macrophages *in vitro* post Mtb infection. Myeloid cell sorting by flow cytometry showed reduced IL-6, IL-1β, IL-10, TGFβ, Nos2, Arg1, Mrc1 and Ym1 in MIR99AHG KD mice compared to the control group. Collectively, these results suggest that MIR99AHG is a target for Mtb for contribution in TB disease progression and increased histopathology.

5.3 Studies contributing to generation of the hypothesis in Chapter 3

Our work followed on from two pivotal studies on the transcriptional landscape of Mtb in M1 (IFNγ) and M2 (IL-4/IL-13) macrophages [147] and redefining the transcriptional regulatory dynamics of M1 (IFNγ) and M2 (IL-4/IL-13) macrophages by CAGE [142]. Briefly, Roy *et al.* [142, 147] identified novel motifs, transcription factors, protein coding and lncRNA genes differentially expressed in M1 (IFNγ), M2 (IL-4/IL-13) and Mtb infected macrophages. From the differentially expressed lncRNAs identified from Roy *et al.*[147], we functionally validated MIR99AHG with *in vivo* and *in vitro* mouse experiments. The findings reported in our study show the novel functional role of MIR99AHG in M2 (IL-4/IL-13) macrophages and during Mtb infection. Previously, functionally validated lncRNAs during Mtb infection have provided an insight into how Mtb is able to target both miRNAs and lncRNAs for persistence within macrophages [64, 66, 68, 100]. *LncRNA-MEG3* was reported to eradicate *M. bovis* BCG in macrophages via autophagy [68]. Recently our group showed that *miR-143* and *miR-365* are both upregulated in M2 (IL-4/IL-13) and in Mtb infected macrophages. They target c-Maf, Bach-1 and Elmo-1 to reduce intracellular Mtb growth [100]. *MicroRNA-27a* was reported to reduce the intracellular survival of Mtb through controlling Ca^{2+}-associated autophagy [197]. Our current study also shows similar results where knockdown of MIR99AHG reduced mycobacterial load in macrophages and in mice due to increased apoptosis. The comparison of our results to other studies is hindered due to very limited research performed on the functional validation of lncRNAs in polarised and/or Mtb infected macrophages.

5.4 Conclusions to Chapter 3

Overall, we showed that lincRNA-MIR99AHG is abundantly expressed in IL-4/IL-13 polarized mouse and human macrophages and downregulated in Mtb infected macrophages. LincRNA-MIR99AHG was shown to regulate inflammatory gene expression in macrophages stimulated with IL-4/IL-13 and infected with Mtb. Knockdown of MIR99AHG in Mtb-infected mice reduced the mycobacterial burden in lung and spleen as well as in macrophages *in vitro*. We report that MIR99AHG regulates the expression of its nearby gene, Cxadr and mediates these functions by interaction with the protein-coding gene hnRNPB2/A1. We show that MIR99AHG is downregulated in PBMCs of active TB patients. We propose a model whereby IL-4/IL-13 induces the upregulation of MIR99AHG which is then targeted by Mtb for intracellular survival in macrophages.

5.5 Aim for chapter 4

The aim of this study was to functionally validate lncRNA IL7-AS in polarized and/or Mtb-infected macrophages using chemically engineered antisense oligonucleotides (GapmeRs). To accomplish this investigation, we performed knockdown experiments of IL7-AS in mice and human macrophages using LNA antisense oligonucleotides known as GapmeRs.

5.6 Summary of results from chapter 4

Our work on the functional role of IL7-AS was presented in Chapter 4. There was no distinct differential expression of IL7-AS in M1 (IFNγ) and M2 (IL-4/IL-13) macrophages. However, IL7-AS was noticeably upregulated by Mtb infection in both M1 (IFNγ) and M2 (IL-4/IL-13) macrophages. These results suggest that IL7-AS is induced by Mtb. Following knockdown of IL7-AS in mouse and human macrophages, we observed reduced intracellular Mtb growth. The reduction in bacterial load was due to increased production of IL-6, IL-12, IL-1α and IL-1β. Nitrite production was induced in LNA GapmeR treated BMDMs while we observed no significant difference in arginase production compared to the control. IL7-AS overlaps with the promoter of IL-7 in antisense. We show on this study that knockdown of IL7-AS enhances IL-7 expression however, IL7-AS functions independently of IL-7 for the promotion of Mtb growth. LPS challenge in mice showed that IL7-AS is induced in the peritoneal fluid, spleen and liver. IL7-AS is induced by TLR 4 and 2 ligands. IL7-AS expression was inhibited the absence of NF-κB, MAPK and Myd88 signalling pathways. These findings suggest that IL7-AS is dependent on these signalling pathways. IL7-AS is conserved in humans as well and our results show that IL7-AS is upregulated in human macrophages post Mtb infection and in PBMCs from active TB patients compared to healthy individuals.

5.7 Studies contributing to generation of the hypothesis in Chapter 4

As previously mentioned above, our work follows the two pivotal studies from Roy *et al.* [142, 147]. IL7-AS was chosen to be functionally validated because it is upregulated by Mtb and has not yet been studied in an Mtb disease model. We functionally validated IL7-AS with *in vitro* mouse experiments. Previous studies have shown that IL7-AS is induced by LPS or IL-1β across different cell types and regulates the production of IL-6 [31]. In our study we also show that IL7-AS is induced by LPS and Mtb infection. Findings presented by Liu *et al.* [182] showed that

IL7-AS promote the expression of proinflammatory genes such as CCL2, CCL5, CCL7 and IL-6 in cells stimulated with LPS. In our study we also show similar results in the induction of IL-6, IL-1α and IL-1β in mouse and human macrophages stimulated with LPS or infected with Mtb. A mechanism was revealed whereby IL7-AS was reported to be dependent on the NF-κB and MAPK signalling pathways [182]. These results are supported by the findings from our study. The authors further show that IL7-AS interacts with p300 to regulate histone acetylation at the promoter regions of their target genes [182]. Further experiments *in vivo* need to be performed to strengthen our findings. It would be interesting to perform an *in vivo* study where we treat mice with IL7-AS ASOs and then infect with Mtb or maybe generate a knockout mouse. This would make our story more compelling and make IL7-AS a potential target for host directed therapy (HDT). Currently, there are no *in vivo* studies on the functional role of IL7-AS during Mtb infection or any other disease model.

5.8 Conclusion to Chapter 4

Overall, we show that IL7-AS is induced by Mtb and LPS. It is an important regulator of proinflammatory genes and a target for Mtb growth. We also show that IL7-AS expression is dependent on NF-κB, MAPK and Myd88 pathways. Altogether, IL7-AS could be a potential target for HDT.

5.9 Relevance of studies and future work

Tuberculosis continues to be the leading infectious disease in the world killing more than 1.5 million people per year [1]. South Africa is one of the countries in the world with the highest burden for TB, TB/HIV and MDR-TB [1]. The current prevention for TB is through the vaccination of children with the bacille Calmette-Guerin (BCG) vaccine [1]. The BCG vaccine does not always protect adults from getting infected with TB. There is increasing drug susceptibility for first line drugs and along with this increasing chances for developing MDR-TB and XDR-TB [1]. New anti-TB therapies that target host factors are needed. Long noncoding RNAs are potential host-derived drug targets which can be used for diagnosing and/or treating tuberculosis. Therapeutics that directly target lncRNAs are promising for many diseases and disorders. Our study was the first line of work which inhibited these lncRNAs in mouse models during Mtb infection. Our results do show these lncRNAs could potentially be used as therapeutics in TB. The next step would be to check the efficacy of these ASOs in a clinical trial. As mentioned previously in the literature review, there is quite a few ASOs that have been approved by the FDA and including the ASOs that are currently in clinical trials for various diseases. Our research group will soon start a clinical trial on simvastatin as host-directed therapy for TB. It is our goal that one of these lncRNAs will one day be involved in a clinical trial as an anti-TB therapeutic.

References

1.   WHO, *Global Tuberculosis Report.* 2019.
2.   Ismail, N.A., et al., *Prevalence of drug-resistant tuberculosis and imputed burden in South Africa: a national and sub-national cross-sectional survey.* Lancet Infect Dis, 2018. **18**(7): p. 779-787.
3.   Guler, R. and F. Brombacher, *Host-directed drug therapy for tuberculosis.* Nat Chem Biol, 2015. **11**(10): p. 748-51.
4.   Deretic, V., et al., *Mycobacterium tuberculosis inhibition of phagolysosome biogenesis and autophagy as a host defence mechanism.* Cell Microbiol, 2006. **8**(5): p. 719-27.
5.   Sturgill-Koszycki, S., et al., *Lack of acidification in Mycobacterium phagosomes produced by exclusion of the vesicular proton-ATPase.* Science, 1994. **263**(5147): p. 678-81.
6.   Malik, Z.A., et al., *Cutting edge: Mycobacterium tuberculosis blocks Ca2+ signaling and phagosome maturation in human macrophages via specific inhibition of sphingosine kinase.* J Immunol, 2003. **170**(6): p. 2811-5.
7.   Fratti, R.A., et al., *Mycobacterium tuberculosis glycosylated phosphatidylinositol causes phagosome maturation arrest.* Proc Natl Acad Sci U S A, 2003. **100**(9): p. 5437-42.
8.   Flynn, J.L. and J. Chan, *Immunology of tuberculosis.* Annu Rev Immunol, 2001. **19**: p. 93-129.
9.   Harrow, J., et al., *GENCODE: the reference human genome annotation for The ENCODE Project.* Genome Res, 2012. **22**(9): p. 1760-74.
10.   Heward, J.A. and M.A. Lindsay, *Long non-coding RNAs in the regulation of the immune response.* Trends Immunol, 2014. **35**(9): p. 408-19.
11.   Maass, P.G., F.C. Luft, and S. Bahring, *Long non-coding RNA in health and disease.* J Mol Med (Berl), 2014. **92**(4): p. 337-46.
12.   Atianand, M.K., D.R. Caffrey, and K.A. Fitzgerald, *Immunobiology of Long Noncoding RNAs.* Annu Rev Immunol, 2017. **35**: p. 177-198.
13.   Atianand, M.K., et al., *A Long Noncoding RNA lincRNA-EPS Acts as a Transcriptional Brake to Restrain Inflammation.* Cell, 2016. **165**(7): p. 1672-85.
14.   Carpenter, S., et al., *A long noncoding RNA mediates both activation and repression of immune response genes.* Science, 2013. **341**(6147): p. 789-92.
15.   Li, Z., et al., *The long noncoding RNA THRIL regulates TNFalpha expression through its interaction with hnRNPL.* Proc Natl Acad Sci U S A, 2014. **111**(3): p. 1002-7.
16.   Du, M., et al., *The LPS-inducible lncRNA Mirt2 is a negative regulator of inflammation.* Nat Commun, 2017. **8**(1): p. 2049.
17.   Castellanos-Rubio, A., et al., *A long noncoding RNA associated with susceptibility to celiac disease.* Science, 2016. **352**(6281): p. 91-5.
18.   Fitzgerald, K.A. and D.R. Caffrey, *Long noncoding RNAs in innate and adaptive immunity.* Curr Opin Immunol, 2014. **26**: p. 140-6.
19.   Katayama, S., et al., *Antisense transcription in the mammalian transcriptome.* Science, 2005. **309**(5740): p. 1564-6.
20.   Zhao, Y., et al., *NONCODE 2016: an informative and valuable data source of long non-coding RNAs.* Nucleic Acids Res, 2016. **44**(D1): p. D203-8.

21.   Geng, H. and X.D. Tan, *Functional diversity of long non-coding RNAs in immune regulation.* Genes Dis, 2016. **3**(1): p. 72-81.

22.   Derrien, T., et al., *The GENCODE v7 catalog of human long noncoding RNAs: analysis of their gene structure, evolution, and expression.* Genome Res, 2012. **22**(9): p. 1775-89.

23.   Djebali, S., et al., *Landscape of transcription in human cells.* Nature, 2012. **489**(7414): p. 101-8.

24.   Ulitsky, I. and D.P. Bartel, *lincRNAs: genomics, evolution, and mechanisms.* Cell, 2013. **154**(1): p. 26-46.

25.   Cabili, M.N., et al., *Integrative annotation of human large intergenic noncoding RNAs reveals global properties and specific subclasses.* Genes Dev, 2011. **25**(18): p. 1915-27.

26.   Kutter, C., et al., *Rapid turnover of long noncoding RNAs and the evolution of gene expression.* PLoS Genet, 2012. **8**(7): p. e1002841.

27.   Necsulea, A., et al., *The evolution of lncRNA repertoires and expression patterns in tetrapods.* Nature, 2014. **505**(7485): p. 635-40.

28.   Geisler, S. and J. Coller, *RNA in unexpected places: long non-coding RNA functions in diverse cellular contexts.* Nat Rev Mol Cell Biol, 2013. **14**(11): p. 699-712.

29.   Emmrich, S., et al., *LincRNAs MONC and MIR100HG act as oncogenes in acute megakaryoblastic leukemia.* Mol Cancer, 2014. **13**: p. 171.

30.   Roux, B., *Catalog of differentially expressed long non-coding RNA following activation of human and mouse innate immune respone.* Frontiers in Immunology, 2017. **8**(1038).

31.   Roux, B.T., et al., *Catalog of Differentially Expressed Long Non-Coding RNA following Activation of Human and Mouse Innate Immune Response.* Front Immunol, 2017. **8**: p. 1038.

32.   Villegas, V.E. and P.G. Zaphiropoulos, *Neighboring gene regulation by antisense long non-coding RNAs.* Int J Mol Sci, 2015. **16**(2): p. 3251-66.

33.   Atkinson, S.R., S. Marguerat, and J. Bahler, *Exploring long non-coding RNAs through sequencing.* Semin Cell Dev Biol, 2012. **23**(2): p. 200-5.

34.   Chen, L.L. and G.G. Carmichael, *Decoding the function of nuclear long non-coding RNAs.* Curr Opin Cell Biol, 2010. **22**(3): p. 357-64.

35.   Dinger, M.E., et al., *Pervasive transcription of the eukaryotic genome: functional indices and conceptual implications.* Brief Funct Genomic Proteomic, 2009. **8**(6): p. 407-23.

36.   Nishizawa, M., et al., *Regulation of inducible gene expression by natural antisense transcripts.* Front Biosci (Landmark Ed), 2012. **17**: p. 938-58.

37.   Clark, B.S. and S. Blackshaw, *Long non-coding RNA-dependent transcriptional regulation in neuronal development and disease.* Front Genet, 2014. **5**: p. 164.

38.   Guttman, M. and J.L. Rinn, *Modular regulatory principles of large non-coding RNAs.* Nature, 2012. **482**(7385): p. 339-46.

39.   Zhang, Y., L. Yang, and L.L. Chen, *Life without A tail: new formats of long noncoding RNAs.* Int J Biochem Cell Biol, 2014. **54**: p. 338-49.

40.   Ilott, N.E. and C.P. Ponting, *Predicting long non-coding RNAs using RNA sequencing.* Methods, 2013. **63**(1): p. 50-9.

41.   Yang, X., et al., *A network based method for analysis of lncRNA-disease associations and prediction of lncRNAs implicated in diseases.* PLoS One, 2014. **9**(1): p. e87797.

42.   Lu, Q., et al., *Computational prediction of associations between long non-coding RNAs and proteins.* BMC Genomics, 2013. **14**: p. 651.

43.   Cui, H., et al., *The human long noncoding RNA lnc-IL7R regulates the inflammatory response.* Eur J Immunol, 2014. **44**(7): p. 2085-95.

44.   NE, I.I., et al., *Long non-coding RNAs and enhancer RNAs regulate the lipopolysaccharide-induced inflammatory response in human monocytes.* Nat Commun, 2014. **5**: p. 3979.

45.   Neguembor, M.V., M. Jothi, and D. Gabellini, *Long noncoding RNAs, emerging players in muscle differentiation and disease.* Skelet Muscle, 2014. **4**(1): p. 8.

46.   Rossetto, C.C., et al., *Regulation of viral and cellular gene expression by Kaposi's sarcoma-associated herpesvirus polyadenylated nuclear RNA.* J Virol, 2013. **87**(10): p. 5540-53.

47.   Gomez, J.A., et al., *The NeST long ncRNA controls microbial susceptibility and epigenetic activation of the interferon-gamma locus.* Cell, 2013. **152**(4): p. 743-54.

48.   Rossetto, C.C. and G. Pari, *KSHV PAN RNA associates with demethylases UTX and JMJD3 to activate lytic replication through a physical interaction with the virus genome.* PLoS Pathog, 2012. **8**(5): p. e1002680.

49.   Zhang, Q., et al., *NEAT1 long noncoding RNA and paraspeckle bodies modulate HIV-1 posttranscriptional expression.* MBio, 2013. **4**(1): p. e00596-12.

50.   Borah, S., et al., *A viral nuclear noncoding RNA binds re-localized poly(A) binding protein and is required for late KSHV gene expression.* PLoS Pathog, 2011. **7**(10): p. e1002300.

51.   Guttman, M., et al., *Chromatin signature reveals over a thousand highly conserved large non-coding RNAs in mammals.* Nature, 2009. **458**(7235): p. 223-7.

52.   Dave, R.K., et al., *Regulated expression of PTPRJ/CD148 and an antisense long noncoding RNA in macrophages by proinflammatory stimuli.* PLoS One, 2013. **8**(6): p. e68306.

53.   Garmire, L.X., et al., *A global clustering algorithm to identify long intergenic non-coding RNA--with applications in mouse macrophages.* PLoS One, 2011. **6**(9): p. e24051.

54.   Peng, X., et al., *Unique signatures of long noncoding RNA expression in response to virus infection and altered innate immune signaling.* MBio, 2010. **1**(5).

55.   Rapicavoli, N.A., et al., *A mammalian pseudogene lncRNA at the interface of inflammation and anti-inflammatory therapeutics.* Elife, 2013. **2**: p. e00762.

56.   Wang, P., et al., *The STAT3-binding long noncoding RNA lnc-DC controls human dendritic cell differentiation.* Science, 2014. **344**(6181): p. 310-3.

57.   Sauvageau, M., et al., *Multiple knockout mouse models reveal lincRNAs are required for life and brain development.* Elife, 2013. **2**: p. e01749.

58.   Elling, R., et al., *Genetic Models Reveal cis and trans Immune-Regulatory Activities for lincRNA-Cox2.* Cell Rep, 2018. **25**(6): p. 1511-1524 e6.

59.   Hu, W., et al., *Long noncoding RNA-mediated anti-apoptotic activity in murine erythroid terminal differentiation.* Genes Dev, 2011. **25**(24): p. 2573-8.

60.   Bold, T.D. and J.D. Ernst, *CD4+ T cell-dependent IFN-gamma production by CD8+ effector T cells in Mycobacterium tuberculosis infection.* J Immunol, 2012. **189**(5): p. 2530-6.

61.   Cooper, A.M., *Cell-mediated immune responses in tuberculosis.* Annu Rev Immunol, 2009. **27**: p. 393-422.

62.   Waggoner, S.N., et al., *Absence of mouse 2B4 promotes NK cell-mediated killing of activated CD8+ T cells, leading to prolonged viral persistence and altered pathogenesis.* J Clin Invest, 2010. **120**(6): p. 1925-38.

63.   Kambayashi, T., et al., *Cutting edge: Regulation of CD8(+) T cell proliferation by 2B4/CD48 interactions.* J Immunol, 2001. **167**(12): p. 6706-10.

64.   Wang, Y., et al., *Long noncoding RNA derived from CD244 signaling epigenetically controls CD8+ T-cell immune responses in tuberculosis infection.* Proc Natl Acad Sci U S A, 2015. **112**(29): p. E3883-92.

65.   Huang, S., et al., *The Expression of lncRNA NEAT1 in Human Tuberculosis and Its Antituberculosis Effect.* Biomed Res Int, 2018. **2018**: p. 9529072.

66.   Li, M., et al., *Long non-coding PCED1B-AS1 regulates macrophage apoptosis and autophagy by sponging miR-155 in active tuberculosis.* Biochemical and Biophysical Research Communications, 2019. **509**(3): p. 803-809.

67.   Ying, L., et al., *Downregulated MEG3 activates autophagy and increases cell proliferation in bladder cancer.* Mol Biosyst, 2013. **9**(3): p. 407-11.

68.   Pawar, K., et al., *Down regulated lncRNA MEG3 eliminates mycobacteria in macrophages via autophagy.* Sci Rep, 2016. **6**: p. 19416.

69.	Chen, W., Yang, X., Zhao, Y., Xu, S., Wang D., *lncRNA-Cox2 enhance the intracellular killing ability against mycobacterium tuberculosis via up-regulating macrophage M1 polarization/nitric oxide production.* 2019.

70.	Hmama, Z., et al., *Immunoevasion and immunosuppression of the macrophage by Mycobacterium tuberculosis.* Immunol Rev, 2015. **264**(1): p. 220-32.

71.	Yang, X., et al., *Microarray analysis of long noncoding RNA and mRNA expression profiles in human macrophages infected with Mycobacterium tuberculosis.* Sci Rep, 2016. **6**: p. 38963.

72.	Yan, H., et al., *Identifying differentially expressed long non-coding RNAs in PBMCs in response to the infection of multidrug-resistant tuberculosis.* Infect Drug Resist, 2018. **11**: p. 945-959.

73.	Chen, Z.L., et al., *Screening and identification of lncRNAs as potential biomarkers for pulmonary tuberculosis.* Sci Rep, 2017. **7**(1): p. 16751.

74.	Yi, Z., et al., *Identifcation of differentially expressed long non-coding RNAs in CD4+ T cells response to latent tuberculosis infection.* J Infect, 2014. **69**(6): p. 558-68.

75.	Butler, A.A., W.M. Webb, and F.D. Lubin, *Regulatory RNAs and control of epigenetic mechanisms: expectations for cognition and cognitive dysfunction.* Epigenomics, 2016. **8**(1): p. 135-51.

76.	Modali, S.D., et al., *Epigenetic regulation of the lncRNA MEG3 and its target c-MET in pancreatic neuroendocrine tumors.* Mol Endocrinol, 2015. **29**(2): p. 224-37.

77.	Peschansky, V.J., et al., *Changes in expression of the long non-coding RNA FMR4 associate with altered gene expression during differentiation of human neural precursor cells.* Front Genet, 2015. **6**: p. 263.

78.	Yan, K., et al., *Structure Prediction: New Insights into Decrypting Long Noncoding RNAs.* Int J Mol Sci, 2016. **17**(1).

79.	Xing, Z., et al., *lncRNA directs cooperative epigenetic regulation downstream of chemokine signals.* Cell, 2014. **159**(5): p. 1110-25.

80.	Wang, K.C., et al., *A long noncoding RNA maintains active chromatin to coordinate homeotic gene expression.* Nature, 2011. **472**(7341): p. 120-4.

81.	Ponting, C.P., P.L. Oliver, and W. Reik, *Evolution and functions of long noncoding RNAs.* Cell, 2009. **136**(4): p. 629-41.

82.	Pandey, R.R., et al., *Kcnq1ot1 antisense noncoding RNA mediates lineage-specific transcriptional silencing through chromatin-level regulation.* Mol Cell, 2008. **32**(2): p. 232-46.

83.	Rinn, J.L., et al., *Functional demarcation of active and silent chromatin domains in human HOX loci by noncoding RNAs.* Cell, 2007. **129**(7): p. 1311-23.

84.	Agostini, F., et al., *X-inactivation: quantitative predictions of protein interactions in the Xist network.* Nucleic Acids Res, 2013. **41**(1): p. e31.

85.	Gupta, R.A., et al., *Long non-coding RNA HOTAIR reprograms chromatin state to promote cancer metastasis.* Nature, 2010. **464**(7291): p. 1071-6.

86.	Jiao, F., et al., *Elevated expression level of long noncoding RNA MALAT-1 facilitates cell growth, migration and invasion in pancreatic cancer.* Oncol Rep, 2014. **32**(6): p. 2485-92.

87.	Faghihi, M.A., et al., *Expression of a noncoding RNA is elevated in Alzheimer's disease and drives rapid feed-forward regulation of beta-secretase.* Nat Med, 2008. **14**(7): p. 723-30.

88.	Novikova, I.V., S.P. Hennelly, and K.Y. Sanbonmatsu, *Tackling structures of long noncoding RNAs.* Int J Mol Sci, 2013. **14**(12): p. 23672-84.

89.	Wan, Y., et al., *Understanding the transcriptome through RNA structure.* Nat Rev Genet, 2011. **12**(9): p. 641-55.

90.	Brion, P. and E. Westhof, *Hierarchy and dynamics of RNA folding.* Annu Rev Biophys Biomol Struct, 1997. **26**: p. 113-37.

91.	Dann, C.E., 3rd, et al., *Structure and mechanism of a metal-sensing regulatory RNA.* Cell, 2007. **130**(5): p. 878-92.

92.	Ashbourne Excoffon, K.J., T. Moninger, and J. Zabner, *The coxsackie B virus and adenovirus receptor resides in a distinct membrane microdomain.* J Virol, 2003. **77**(4): p. 2559-67.

93.   Giaginis, C.T., et al., *Coxsackievirus and adenovirus receptor expression in human endometrial adenocarcinoma: possible clinical implications.* World J Surg Oncol, 2008. **6**: p. 59.

94.   Excoffon, K.J., et al., *A role for the PDZ-binding domain of the coxsackie B virus and adenovirus receptor (CAR) in cell adhesion and growth.* J Cell Sci, 2004. **117**(Pt 19): p. 4401-9.

95.   Jin, W. and C. Dong, *IL-17 cytokines in immunity and inflammation.* Emerg Microbes Infect, 2013. **2**(9): p. e60.

96.   Zhong, B., et al., *Negative regulation of IL-17-mediated signaling and inflammation by the ubiquitin-specific protease USP25.* Nat Immunol, 2012. **13**(11): p. 1110-7.

97.   Wu, J., et al., *Analysis of microRNA expression profiling identifies miR-155 and miR-155* as potential diagnostic markers for active tuberculosis: a preliminary study.* Hum Immunol, 2012. **73**(1): p. 31-7.

98.   Kumar, R., et al., *Identification of a novel role of ESAT-6-dependent miR-155 induction during infection of macrophages with Mycobacterium tuberculosis.* Cell Microbiol, 2012. **14**(10): p. 1620-31.

99.   Singh, P.K., A.V. Singh, and D.S. Chauhan, *Current understanding on micro RNAs and its regulation in response to Mycobacterial infections.* J Biomed Sci, 2013. **20**: p. 14.

100.   Tamgue, O., et al., *Differential Targeting of c-Maf, Bach-1, and Elmo-1 by microRNA-143 and microRNA-365 Promotes the Intracellular Growth of Mycobacterium tuberculosis in Alternatively IL-4/IL-13 Activated Macrophages.* Front Immunol, 2019. **10**: p. 421.

101.   Majid, S., et al., *BTG3 tumor suppressor gene promoter demethylation, histone modification and cell cycle arrest by genistein in renal cancer.* Carcinogenesis, 2009. **30**(4): p. 662-70.

102.   Ou, Y.H., et al., *The candidate tumor suppressor BTG3 is a transcriptional target of p53 that inhibits E2F1.* EMBO J, 2007. **26**(17): p. 3968-80.

103.   Rahmani, Z., *APRO4 negatively regulates Src tyrosine kinase activity in PC12 cells.* J Cell Sci, 2006. **119**(Pt 4): p. 646-58.

104.   Yamamoto, N., et al., *Analysis of the ANA gene as a candidate for the chromosome 21q oral cancer susceptibility locus.* Br J Cancer, 2001. **84**(6): p. 754-9.

105.   Young, C., G. Walzl, and N. Du Plessis, *Therapeutic host-directed strategies to improve outcome in tuberculosis.* Mucosal Immunol, 2020. **13**(2): p. 190-204.

106.   WHO, *Global tuberculosis report* WHO, 2019.

107.   Wallis, R.S. and R. Hafner, *Advancing host-directed therapy for tuberculosis.* Nat Rev Immunol, 2015. **15**(4): p. 255-63.

108.   Cohen, S.P., et al., *Randomized, double-blind, comparative-effectiveness study comparing pulsed radiofrequency to steroid injections for occipital neuralgia or migraine with occipital nerve tenderness.* Pain, 2015. **156**(12): p. 2585-94.

109.   de Gans, J., D. van de Beek, and I. European Dexamethasone in Adulthood Bacterial Meningitis Study, *Dexamethasone in adults with bacterial meningitis.* N Engl J Med, 2002. **347**(20): p. 1549-56.

110.   Schutz, C., et al., *Corticosteroids as an adjunct to tuberculosis therapy.* Expert Rev Respir Med, 2018. **12**(10): p. 881-891.

111.   *PREDNISOLONE in the treatment of pulmonary tuberculosis: a controlled trial; a preliminary report by the Research Committee of the Tuberculosis Society of Scotland.* Br Med J, 1957. **2**(5054): p. 1131-4.

112.   Dooley, D.P., J.L. Carpenter, and S. Rademacher, *Adjunctive corticosteroid therapy for tuberculosis: a critical reappraisal of the literature.* Clin Infect Dis, 1997. **25**(4): p. 872-87.

113.   Lavers, K.W. and J.C. Roberts, *The use of prednisone in primary tuberculosis in children.* Tubercle, 1959. **40**: p. 173-6.

114.   Meintjes, G., et al., *Randomized placebo-controlled trial of prednisone for paradoxical tuberculosis-associated immune reconstitution inflammatory syndrome.* AIDS, 2010. **24**(15): p. 2381-90.

115.   Singhal, A., et al., *Metformin as adjunct antituberculosis therapy.* Sci Transl Med, 2014. **6**(263): p. 263ra159.

116.   Dutta, N.K., et al., *Adjunctive Host-Directed Therapy With Statins Improves Tuberculosis-Related Outcomes in Mice.* J Infect Dis, 2020. **221**(7): p. 1079-1087.

117.   Parihar, S.P., et al., *Statin therapy reduces the mycobacterium tuberculosis burden in human macrophages and in mice by enhancing autophagy and phagosome maturation.* J Infect Dis, 2014. **209**(5): p. 754-63.

118.   Mily, A., et al., *Significant Effects of Oral Phenylbutyrate and Vitamin D3 Adjunctive Therapy in Pulmonary Tuberculosis: A Randomized Controlled Trial.* PLoS One, 2015. **10**(9): p. e0138340.

119.   Schiebler, M., et al., *Functional drug screening reveals anticonvulsants as enhancers of mTOR-independent autophagic killing of Mycobacterium tuberculosis through inositol depletion.* EMBO Mol Med, 2015. **7**(2): p. 127-39.

120.   Bajan, S. and G. Hutvagner, *RNA-Based Therapeutics: From Antisense Oligonucleotides to miRNAs.* Cells, 2020. **9**(1).

121.   Chan, J.H., S. Lim, and W.S. Wong, *Antisense oligonucleotides: from design to therapeutic application.* Clin Exp Pharmacol Physiol, 2006. **33**(5-6): p. 533-40.

122.   Chery, J., *RNA therapeutics: RNAi and antisense mechanisms and clinical applications.* Postdoc J, 2016. **4**(7): p. 35-50.

123.   Di Fusco, D., et al., *Antisense Oligonucleotide: Basic Concepts and Therapeutic Application in Inflammatory Bowel Disease.* Front Pharmacol, 2019. **10**: p. 305.

124.   Bennett, C.F., et al., *Pharmacology of Antisense Drugs.* Annu Rev Pharmacol Toxicol, 2017. **57**: p. 81-105.

125.   Crooke, S.T., *Molecular Mechanisms of Antisense Oligonucleotides.* Nucleic Acid Ther, 2017. **27**(2): p. 70-77.

126.   Scoles, D.R. and S.M. Pulst, *Oligonucleotide therapeutics in neurodegenerative diseases.* RNA Biol, 2018. **15**(6): p. 707-714.

127.   Andronescu, M., Z.C. Zhang, and A. Condon, *Secondary structure prediction of interacting RNA molecules.* J Mol Biol, 2005. **345**(5): p. 987-1001.

128.   Ho, S.P., et al., *Mapping of RNA accessible sites for antisense experiments with oligonucleotide libraries.* Nat Biotechnol, 1998. **16**(1): p. 59-63.

129.   Vickers, T.A., J.R. Wyatt, and S.M. Freier, *Effects of RNA secondary structure on cellular antisense activity.* Nucleic Acids Res, 2000. **28**(6): p. 1340-7.

130.   Eckstein, F., *Phosphorothioates, essential components of therapeutic oligonucleotides.* Nucleic Acid Ther, 2014. **24**(6): p. 374-87.

131.   Eder, P.S., et al., *Substrate specificity and kinetics of degradation of antisense oligonucleotides by a 3' exonuclease in plasma.* Antisense Res Dev, 1991. **1**(2): p. 141-51.

132.   Soutschek, J., et al., *Therapeutic silencing of an endogenous gene by systemic administration of modified siRNAs.* Nature, 2004. **432**(7014): p. 173-8.

133.   Tahara, K., W. Hashimoto, and H. Takeuchi, *Inhalation Properties and Stability of Nebulized Naked siRNA Solution for Pulmonary Therapy.* Chem Pharm Bull (Tokyo), 2016. **64**(1): p. 63-7.

134.   Deng, Y., et al., *Transdermal Delivery of siRNA through Microneedle Array.* Sci Rep, 2016. **6**: p. 21422.

135.   Jabs, D.A. and P.D. Griffiths, *Fomivirsen for the treatment of cytomegalovirus retinitis.* Am J Ophthalmol, 2002. **133**(4): p. 552-6.

136.   Duell, P.B., et al., *Long-term mipomersen treatment is associated with a reduction in cardiovascular events in patients with familial hypercholesterolemia.* J Clin Lipidol, 2016. **10**(4): p. 1011-1021.

137.   Khorkova, O. and C. Wahlestedt, *Oligonucleotide therapies for disorders of the nervous system.* Nat Biotechnol, 2017. **35**(3): p. 249-263.

138. Goyal, N. and P. Narayanaswami, *Making sense of antisense oligonucleotides: A narrative review.* Muscle Nerve, 2018. **57**(3): p. 356-370.

139. Stein, C., et al., *Defibrotide (Defitelio): A New Addition to the Stockpile of Food and Drug Administration-approved Oligonucleotide Drugs.* Mol Ther Nucleic Acids, 2016. **5**: p. e346.

140. Lawrance, I.C., et al., *A murine model of chronic inflammation-induced intestinal fibrosis down-regulated by antisense NF-kappa B.* Gastroenterology, 2003. **125**(6): p. 1750-61.

141. Feagan, B.G., et al., *Effects of Mongersen (GED-0301) on Endoscopic and Clinical Outcomes in Patients With Active Crohn's Disease.* Gastroenterology, 2018. **154**(1): p. 61-64 e6.

142. Roy, S., et al., *Redefining the transcriptional regulatory dynamics of classically and alternatively activated macrophages by deepCAGE transcriptomics.* Nucleic Acids Res, 2015. **43**(14): p. 6969-82.

143. Heyer, E.E., et al., *An optimized kit-free method for making strand-specific deep sequencing libraries from RNA fragments.* Nucleic Acids Res, 2015. **43**(1): p. e2.

144. Guler, R., et al., *IL-4Ralpha-dependent alternative activation of macrophages is not decisive for Mycobacterium tuberculosis pathology and bacterial burden in mice.* PLoS One, 2015. **10**(3): p. e0121070.

145. Elling, R., J. Chan, and K.A. Fitzgerald, *Emerging role of long noncoding RNAs as regulators of innate immune cell development and inflammatory gene expression.* Eur J Immunol, 2016. **46**(3): p. 504-12.

146. Penny, G.D., et al., *Requirement for Xist in X chromosome inactivation.* Nature, 1996. **379**(6561): p. 131-7.

147. Roy, S., et al., *Transcriptional landscape of Mycobacterium tuberculosis infection in macrophages.* Sci Rep, 2018. **8**(1): p. 6758.

148. Iannaccone, M., A. Dorhoi, and S.H. Kaufmann, *Host-directed therapy of tuberculosis: what is in it for microRNA?* Expert Opin Ther Targets, 2014. **18**(5): p. 491-4.

149. Man, D.K., et al., *Potential and development of inhaled RNAi therapeutics for the treatment of pulmonary tuberculosis.* Adv Drug Deliv Rev, 2016. **102**: p. 21-32.

150. Kawasaki, T. and T. Kawai, *Toll-like receptor signaling pathways.* Front Immunol, 2014. **5**: p. 461.

151. Heller, N.M., et al., *IL-4 engagement of the type I IL-4 receptor complex enhances mouse eosinophil migration to eotaxin-1 in vitro.* PLoS One, 2012. **7**(6): p. e39673.

152. Hawn, T.R., et al., *Host-directed therapeutics for tuberculosis: can we harness the host?* Microbiol Mol Biol Rev, 2013. **77**(4): p. 608-27.

153. MacMicking, J.D., et al., *Identification of nitric oxide synthase as a protective locus against tuberculosis.* Proc Natl Acad Sci U S A, 1997. **94**(10): p. 5243-8.

154. O'Connell, R.M., D.S. Rao, and D. Baltimore, *microRNA regulation of inflammatory responses.* Annu Rev Immunol, 2012. **30**: p. 295-312.

155. Behar, S.M., et al., *Apoptosis is an innate defense function of macrophages against Mycobacterium tuberculosis.* Mucosal Immunol, 2011. **4**(3): p. 279-87.

156. Chen, M., H. Gan, and H.G. Remold, *A mechanism of virulence: virulent Mycobacterium tuberculosis strain H37Rv, but not attenuated H37Ra, causes significant mitochondrial inner membrane disruption in macrophages leading to necrosis.* J Immunol, 2006. **176**(6): p. 3707-16.

157. Cooper, A.M., K.D. Mayer-Barber, and A. Sher, *Role of innate cytokines in mycobacterial infection.* Mucosal Immunol, 2011. **4**(3): p. 252-60.

158. Zhang, Q., et al., *The long noncoding RNA ROCKI regulates inflammatory gene expression.* EMBO J, 2019.

159. Yan, R., et al., *The PDZ3 domain of the cellular scaffolding protein MAGI-1 interacts with the Coxsackievirus and adenovirus receptor (CAR).* Int J Biochem Cell Biol, 2015. **61**: p. 29-34.

160. Imamura, K., et al., *Long noncoding RNA NEAT1-dependent SFPQ relocation from promoter region to paraspeckle mediates IL8 expression upon immune stimuli.* Mol Cell, 2014. **53**(3): p. 393-406.

161. Engreitz, J.M., et al., *Local regulation of gene expression by lncRNA promoters, transcription and splicing.* Nature, 2016. **539**(7629): p. 452-455.

162. Guil, S. and M. Esteller, *Cis-acting noncoding RNAs: friends and foes.* Nat Struct Mol Biol, 2012. **19**(11): p. 1068-75.

163. Kopp, F. and J.T. Mendell, *Functional Classification and Experimental Dissection of Long Noncoding RNAs.* Cell, 2018. **172**(3): p. 393-407.

164. Cooper, A.M., *Mouse model of tuberculosis.* Cold Spring Harb Perspect Med, 2014. **5**(2): p. a018556.

165. Zhan, L., et al., *Animal Models for Tuberculosis in Translational and Precision Medicine.* Front Microbiol, 2017. **8**: p. 717.

166. Feyder, M. and L.A. Goff, *Investigating long noncoding RNAs using animal models.* J Clin Invest, 2016. **126**(8): p. 2783-91.

167. Kim, J.K., et al., *MicroRNA in innate immunity and autophagy during mycobacterial infection.* Cell Microbiol, 2017. **19**(1).

168. Yang, T. and B. Ge, *miRNAs in immune responses to Mycobacterium tuberculosis infection.* Cancer Lett, 2018. **431**: p. 22-30.

169. Huarte, M., et al., *A large intergenic noncoding RNA induced by p53 mediates global gene repression in the p53 response.* Cell, 2010. **142**(3): p. 409-19.

170. Hasegawa, Y., et al., *The matrix protein hnRNP U is required for chromosomal localization of Xist RNA.* Dev Cell, 2010. **19**(3): p. 469-76.

171. Hu, J., et al., *Promoter-associated small double-stranded RNA interacts with heterogeneous nuclear ribonucleoprotein A2/B1 to induce transcriptional activation.* Biochem J, 2012. **447**(3): p. 407-16.

172. Wang, G., et al., *Functional impact of heterogeneous nuclear ribonucleoprotein A2/B1 in smooth muscle differentiation from stem cells and embryonic arteriogenesis.* J Biol Chem, 2012. **287**(4): p. 2896-906.

173. Zhang, K., et al., *The ways of action of long non-coding RNAs in cytoplasm and nucleus.* Gene, 2014. **547**(1): p. 1-9.

174. Kotzin, J.J., et al., *The long non-coding RNA Morrbid regulates Bim and short-lived myeloid cell lifespan.* Nature, 2016. **537**(7619): p. 239-243.

175. Huang, W., et al., *DDX5 and its associated lncRNA Rmrp modulate TH17 cell effector functions.* Nature, 2015. **528**(7583): p. 517-22.

176. Zgheib, C., et al., *Long non-coding RNA Lethe regulates hyperglycemia-induced reactive oxygen species production in macrophages.* PLoS One, 2017. **12**(5): p. e0177453.

177. Kumar, H., T. Kawai, and S. Akira, *Pathogen recognition by the innate immune system.* Int Rev Immunol, 2011. **30**(1): p. 16-34.

178. Okazaki, Y., et al., *Analysis of the mouse transcriptome based on functional annotation of 60,770 full-length cDNAs.* Nature, 2002. **420**(6915): p. 563-73.

179. Hadjicharalambous, M.R. and M.A. Lindsay, *Long Non-Coding RNAs and the Innate Immune Response.* Noncoding RNA, 2019. **5**(2).

180. Mathy, N.W. and X.M. Chen, *Long non-coding RNAs (lncRNAs) and their transcriptional control of inflammatory responses.* J Biol Chem, 2017. **292**(30): p. 12375-12382.

181. Ilott, N.E., et al., *Corrigendum: Long non-coding RNAs and enhancer RNAs regulate the lipopolysaccharide-induced inflammatory response in human monocytes.* Nat Commun, 2015. **6**: p. 6814.

182. Liu, X., et al., *A Long Noncoding RNA, Antisense IL-7, Promotes Inflammatory Gene Transcription through Facilitating Histone Acetylation and Switch/Sucrose Nonfermentable Chromatin Remodeling.* J Immunol, 2019. **203**(6): p. 1548-1559.

183.	Niu, N. and X. Qin, *New insights into IL-7 signaling pathways during early and late T cell development.* Cell Mol Immunol, 2013. **10**(3): p. 187-9.

184.	Krawczyk, M. and B.M. Emerson, *p50-associated COX-2 extragenic RNA (PACER) activates COX-2 gene expression by occluding repressive NF-kappaB complexes.* Elife, 2014. **3**: p. e01776.

185.	Bourigault, M.L., et al., *Relative contribution of IL-1alpha, IL-1beta and TNF to the host response to Mycobacterium tuberculosis and attenuated M. bovis BCG.* Immun Inflamm Dis, 2013. **1**(1): p. 47-62.

186.	Nagabhushanam, V., et al., *Innate inhibition of adaptive immunity: Mycobacterium tuberculosis-induced IL-6 inhibits macrophage responses to IFN-gamma.* J Immunol, 2003. **171**(9): p. 4750-7.

187.	Martinez, A.N., S. Mehra, and D. Kaushal, *Role of interleukin 6 in innate immunity to Mycobacterium tuberculosis infection.* J Infect Dis, 2013. **207**(8): p. 1253-61.

188.	ElKassar, N. and R.E. Gress, *An overview of IL-7 biology and its use in immunotherapy.* J Immunotoxicol, 2010. **7**(1): p. 1-7.

189.	Hong, C., M.A. Luckey, and J.H. Park, *Intrathymic IL-7: the where, when, and why of IL-7 signaling during T cell development.* Semin Immunol, 2012. **24**(3): p. 151-8.

190.	Pellegrini, M., et al., *Adjuvant IL-7 antagonizes multiple cellular and molecular inhibitory networks to enhance immunotherapies.* Nat Med, 2009. **15**(5): p. 528-36.

191.	Standiford, T.J., et al., *IL-7 up-regulates the expression of IL-8 from resting and stimulated human blood monocytes.* J Immunol, 1992. **149**(6): p. 2035-9.

192.	Gessner, A., et al., *Interleukin-7 enhances antimicrobial activity against Leishmania major in murine macrophages.* Infect Immun, 1993. **61**(9): p. 4008-12.

193.	Maeurer, M.J., et al., *Interleukin-7 or interleukin-15 enhances survival of Mycobacterium tuberculosis-infected mice.* Infect Immun, 2000. **68**(5): p. 2962-70.

194.	Jo, E.K., et al., *Intracellular signalling cascades regulating innate immune responses to Mycobacteria: branching out from Toll-like receptors.* Cell Microbiol, 2007. **9**(5): p. 1087-98.

195.	Wang, T., W.P. Lafuse, and B.S. Zwilling, *NFkappaB and Sp1 elements are necessary for maximal transcription of toll-like receptor 2 induced by Mycobacterium avium.* J Immunol, 2001. **167**(12): p. 6924-32.

196.	Yadav, M., L. Clark, and J.S. Schorey, *Macrophage's proinflammatory response to a mycobacterial infection is dependent on sphingosine kinase-mediated activation of phosphatidylinositol phospholipase C, protein kinase C, ERK1/2, and phosphatidylinositol 3-kinase.* J Immunol, 2006. **176**(9): p. 5494-503.

197.	Liu, F., et al., *MicroRNA-27a controls the intracellular survival of Mycobacterium tuberculosis by regulating calcium-associated autophagy.* Nat Commun, 2018. **9**(1): p. 4295.